Renal Meal Plan For Kidney Patients

Benjamin C. Murphy

Introduction

This is a comprehensive guide that focuses on dietary recommendations and recipes tailored to individuals with renal issues. It emphasizes the importance of making informed choices to support kidney health.

The guide introduces the renal diet, which is characterized by specific dietary guidelines to manage kidney-related conditions effectively. Key principles of the renal diet include limiting sodium and salt intake, selecting the right types of proteins, consuming foods and drinks low in phosphorus, prioritizing heart-healthy foods, reducing potassium consumption, and monitoring fluid intake.

Benefits of following the renal diet are discussed, highlighting how it can positively impact kidney health and overall well-being.

The cookbook section offers a wide range of recipes suitable for individuals on the renal diet. These recipes are categorized into breakfast options, smoothies, snacks, sides, soups, salads, poultry and meat mains, fish and seafood dishes, and desserts. Each recipe is thoughtfully designed to align with the dietary requirements of renal patients while maintaining delicious and satisfying flavors.

The guide also provides conversion tables for easy reference, making it convenient for readers to adapt recipes to their specific needs.

In summary, this book offers valuable insights into the renal diet and provides a variety of flavorful recipes to support kidney health. It serves as a practical resource for individuals looking to make positive dietary changes in managing renal conditions.

Contents

THE RENAL DIET

As kidney activity is affected, the kidneys do not adequately remove or extract debris. It will adversely influence the electrolyte levels of a patient if the excess is left in the blood. It can even help improve kidney function and delay total kidney disease development by maintaining a kidney diet.

An integral aspect of every recovery regimen for a chronic kidney disorder is a healthy renal diet. One that is low in protein, phosphorous, sodium is a renal diet. A renal diet often highlights the value of eating high-quality protein and typically limiting liquid. Potassium and calcium will also need to be restricted to certain patients. The body of an individual is different, so it is important for each patient to collaborate with a renal dietitian to create a diet customized to the patient's needs. When you have serious kidney failure, you ought to have a kidney-friendly meal schedule. It can encourage you to be healthier by monitoring what you consume and drink.

Your well-being is influenced by what you consume and drink. It will help regulate your blood pressure and keep at a healthier weight and consume a nutritious diet low in salt and fat. You have to regulate your blood pressure if you have diabetes by consciously deciding what you consume and drink. A renal diet can help keep kidney disease from getting worse by managing high blood pressure and diabetes.

Depending on the level of kidney failure, how strict the meal schedule can be. You could have few to no limitations on what you consume and drink in the early stages of kidney disease. Your doctor may consider restricting your:

- Sodium
- Potassium
- Phosphorus

- Protein
- Fluids; If your kidney disease worsens.

Consume Foods with Less Sodium & Salt

Usually, there is a sodium reduction in the context of "No Added Salt." This is important because higher sodium consumption can result in improperly regulated blood pressure and increased thirst, which may contribute to difficulties adhering to your diet's fluid restrictions.

To reduce your sodium intake, you should not consume

- Table salt or any flavoring that has salt in it
- Salt alternative as they can have potassium in them
- Salty meats such as ham, bacon, hot dogs, sausage, bologna, lunch meats, and canned meats,
- Salty snacks such as salted crackers, cheese curls, Chips, salted nuts
- Thoroughly wash canned meats, vegetables, fish, and beans
- Do not eat instant noodles, canned soups, and frozen dinners
- Consume fresh food often.
- Cook foods at home instead of dining out, frozen dinners, canned foods, and fast foods it is better to control ingredients when you make food yourself
- Use sodium-free seasonings, spices, and herbs, instead of salt
- Do not consume brined olives, sauces, MSG, and bottled pickles

Consume The Right Types of Proteins

To help in the development and preservation of body tissue, protein is necessary. Protein also serves a part in the battle against bacteria, wound healing, and allowing the body to supply energy. Per day, you can make sure to consume 7-8 ounces of protein. Protein-rich foods are meat, pork, turkey, beef, and chicken.

Fish, eggs, and seafood. One egg is equivalent to one ounce of protein; 3 ounces of protein is similar to a deck of cards in size. Eat small portions of protein foods on a renal diet

A cooked portion of fish, chicken, or meat is near 2-3 ounces, like to size of a deck of cards. A portion of dairy is one slice of cheese or half a cup of yogurt or milk.

Plant based-protein foods:

- Grains
- Nuts
- Beans

Cooked beans' portion is about half cup. A portion of cooked noodles or cooked rice is a half-cup. A serving of bread is a single slice.

Consume Drinks & Food with Less Phosphorus

Try to eat less of high phosphorus foods like:

- Dairy, Meats, fish, and poultry (you can eat one serving)
- Dairy products Milk and cheese (one 4 oz. serving)
- Avoid this food or eat very less of
  - Black Beans, Lima Beans, Red Beans, White Beans, and Black-eyed Peas
  - Unrefined, Dark, whole grains
  - Refrigerated doughs
  - Vegetables and fruits that are Dried
  - Dark-colored sodas
  - Chocolate

You may take a phosphate binder if prescribed by your doctor. Choose those meats, fish, and pasta that are low in phosphorous. The daily limit is 1000mg/day.

Choose Heart-Healthy Foods

Rather than deep-frying, broil, grill, bake, stir-fry roast, foods. Rather than butter, cook with cooking spray or a tiny quantity of olive oil. Cut fat from meat before eating, remove the skin from the meat. Try to restrict trans fats and saturated fats and Read the nutrients of the food. Low-fat or fat-free milk, yogurt, and cheese

Consume Food with Less Amount of Potassium

High potassium may induce erratic heart rhythms, and if potassium levels get high, it may also cause the heart to stop. For those with a large amount of potassium, there are usually no signs. If Your potassium level is troubling, consult with your doctor
Patients can consume 2000 mg/day of potassium.
Foods that are Lower in Potassium
Peaches, apples, White pasta and bread, Carrots, Rice milk, green beans
White rice, Apple, or grape or cranberry juice, Cooked rice, grits, and wheat cereals.

Limit Intake of Fluids

Your doctor can tell you to restrict the amount of fluid based on kidney disease and recovery levels. You will have to ease up as to how much you drink fluids. Any items that include a lot of water will even need to be cut down on. There is a lot of water in soups or melting items, such as ice, ice cream, and gelatin. Many vegetables and fruits and even have strong water content too.
The daily limit is usually four cups of fluid each day for server kidney failure. or as your doctor has prescribed

There are many benefits to adapting to the renal diet, whether or not you have kidney disease or related conditions. It's a good way to eat and live, especially if you may be susceptible to kidney infections and other issues that impact the function of this vital organ. This includes making changes early and paying close attention to your symptoms and any changes you notice, as these may indicate the progression in the disease itself or a positive change in your kidneys' function. Keeping an eye on the slightest changes can make a significant difference in improving your health and taking charge of your well-being.

The Major Benefits of the Renal Diet

How Eating Well Can Make a Difference

The renal diet focuses primarily on supporting kidney health because, in doing so, you'll improve many other aspects of your health, as well. Preventing the later stages is the main goal, though reaching this stage can still be treated with careful consideration of your dietary choices. In addition to medical treatment, the diet provides a way for you to gain control over your own health and progression. It can mean the difference between a complete renal failure or a manageable chronic condition, where you can lead a regular, enjoyable life despite having kidney issues.

Eating Well is a Natural and Medicine-Free Way to Help Your Kidneys

Whether or not the medication is a part of your treatment plan, your diet takes on a significant role in the health of your kidneys. Some herbs and vitamins can boost the medicinal properties found in foods and give your kidneys additional support while limiting other ingredients, which, in excess, can lead to complete renal failure if there are already signs of kidney impairment. Your kidneys thrive on fresh, unprocessed foods that make it easier for your body to break down, digest, and process nutrients. Choosing natural options also eliminates or reduces the amount of Sodium and refined sugars you consume, so you don't have to continuously monitor how many grams of salt or sugar is in your foods.

If you have limited access to fresh fruits or vegetables, choose frozen as the next best option, as they will have retained all or most of the nutrients in their original state. Canned vegetables and fruits are often processed, though these can be added when no other options are available. To reduce the amount of Sodium they contain, rinse canned vegetables in the water at least twice before adding them to your meal or dish. Canned fruit is often preserved in a thick or sugary syrup, which should be drained and rinsed before serving to reduce the sugar content. Always read the ingredients of the package or can before you consider adding it to your grocery cart, and only choose these options where fresh or frozen selections are unavailable.

Unless directed by a physician or medical specialist, don't reduce or stop taking medication for your kidneys, even if there are significant improvements to your health as a result of dietary changes and/or medical improvements, and there is an increase in kidney function noted. While diet should be a central part of your lifestyle, keep the medication as part of this treatment goal just the same. Any sudden or significant changes in your treatment plan can thwart any progress made and may cause further damage in the long term. Consider your food and meal choices in the renal diet as part of a whole, which also includes exercise, medical treatment(s), and living well.

1. Buttermilk Pancakes

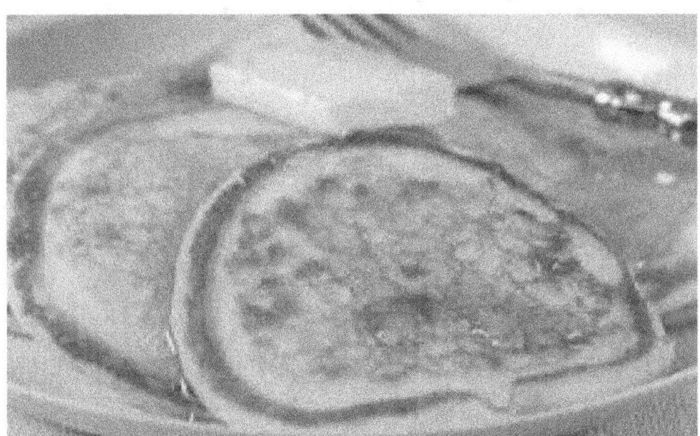

Preparation Time: 10 minutes
Cooking Time: 20 minutes
Servings: 2

Ingredients

- ½ cup almond flour
- ¼ teaspoon cream of tartar
- ½ teaspoons baking soda
- ½ tablespoons honey
- ½ cups low-fat buttermilk
- 1 egg
- ¼ tablespoon olive oil

Directions

1. Warm up a skillet on medium heat.
2. Combine dry ingredients in a large bowl. Add dry ingredients to buttermilk, oil and egg mixture. Use a whisk or spoon to blend the dry ingredients until they are completely moist. Use a teaspoon of olive oil to grease the skillet. Using a 1/3-cup measuring cup, scoop the pancake

mixture on the skillet. Each pancake should spread to about 4 inches across. Leave about 2 inches between the pancakes for easy flipping. Flip pancakes using a spatula —do this when the bubbles on the top of the pancakes have mostly disappeared. Allow the other side to brown until the center no longer appears wet.

3. Move to a serving dish.
4. For a healthier twist, think of serving with fresh berries and a side of eggs.

NutritionCalories: 124 Total Fat: 9.2g Saturated Fat: 1.1g Cholesterol: 42mg Sodium: 206mg Total Carbohydrate: 6.8g Protein: 5.4g Potassium: 94mg Phosphorus: 80mg

2. Egg Pockets

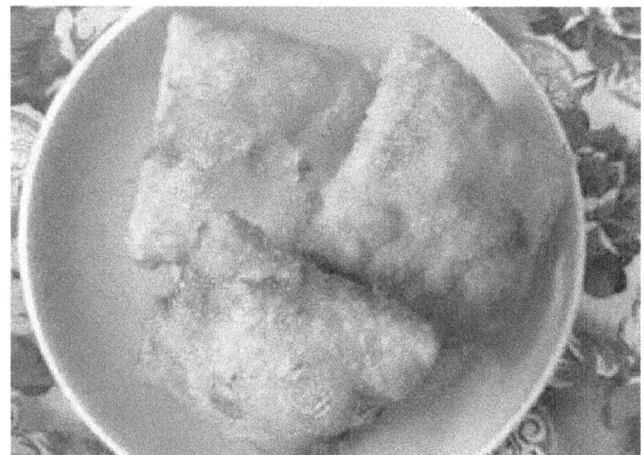

Preparation Time: 10 minutes
Cooking Time: 15 minutes
Servings: 2
Ingredients

- ¼ teaspoons dry yeast
- 1 cup warm water
- 1 tablespoon olive oil
- 1 tablespoon honey

- 1 garlic clove, minced
- ½ cup almond flour
- 1 egg
- ½ tablespoon cream cheese

Directions

1. Dissolve yeast in warm water. Stir in olive oil, honey, minced garlic, and almond flour to make a soft dough. Place in a greased bowl, cover and set aside. Let rest 5 minutes. Roll dough out to 1/2-inch thickness. Cut into 4 pieces. Scramble eggs and stir in cream cheese. Place egg mixture onto 1/2 of each piece of dough. Fold dough over, pinching edges, then cut top to vent.
2. Spray top of each pocket with oil
3. Bake at 350°F for 15 to 20 minutes, until light golden brown.

NutritionCalories: 150 Total Fat: 12.1g Cholesterol: 42mg Sodium: 22mg Total Carbohydrate: 8.1g Protein: 4.9g Calcium: 41mg Iron: 1mg Potassium: 43mg Phosphorus: 35mg

3. Omelets with Vegetables

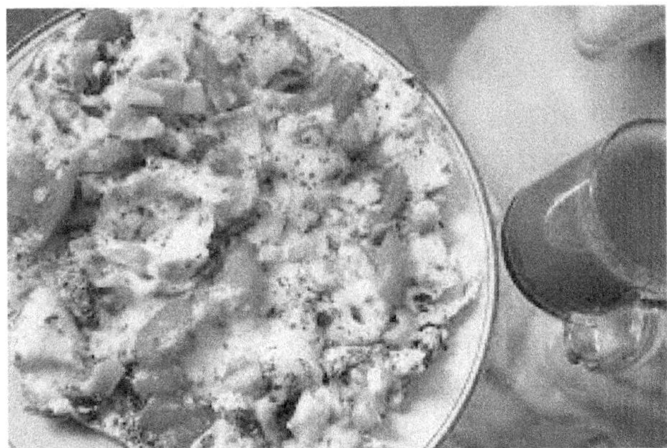

Preparation Time: 10 minutes

Cooking Time: 15 minutes
Servings: 2
Ingredients

- 1/8 cup zucchini, chopped
- 1/8 cup red bell pepper, chopped
- 1/8 cup kale, chopped
- 3 tablespoons green onion, chopped
- 2 tablespoons water
- 1/4 teaspoon dried dill
- 2 large egg whites
- 1-ounce low-fat sharp parmesan cheese, shredded
- ¼ tablespoon olive oil

Directions

1. Heat a small saucepan over medium-high heat. Coat pan with oil. Add bell pepper, zucchini, kale and onions to pan; sauté 4 minutes or until vegetables are crisp-tender. Remove from heat.
2. Heat a 10-inch non-stick skillet over medium-high heat. Combine water, pepper, dill, and egg whites in a bowl, stirring well with a whisk.
3. Coat pan with cooking spray. Pour egg mixture into pan; cook until edges begin to set (about 2 minutes). Gently lift the edges of the omelet with a spatula, tilting the pan to allow uncooked egg mixture to come into contact with the pan.
4. Spoon vegetable mixture onto half of omelet, sprinkle cheese over vegetable mixture. Loosen omelet with a spatula and fold in half. Cook 2 minutes more or until cheese melts. Carefully slide omelet onto a plate.

Nutrition: Calories: 85 Total Fat: 4g Saturated Fat: 2.5g Cholesterol: 10mg Sodium: 278mg Total Carbohydrate: 2.7g Protein: 9.5g Calcium: 196mg Iron: 0mg Potassium: 150mg Phosphorus: 118mg

4. Sausage Breakfast Sandwich

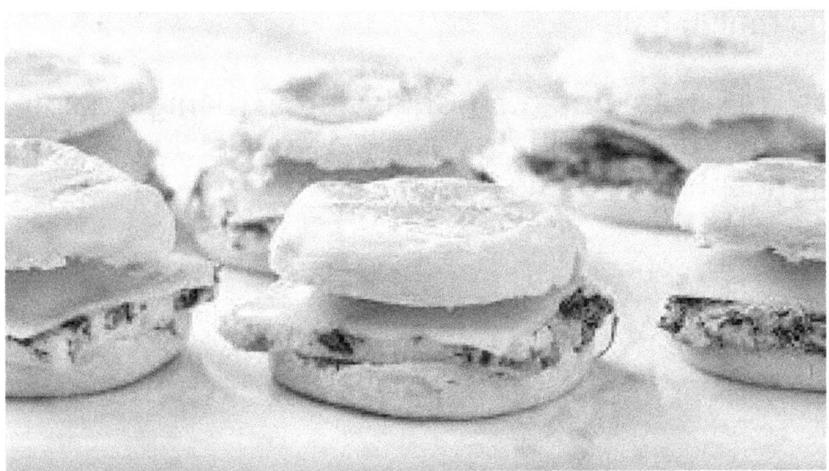

Preparation Time: 10 minutes
Cooking Time: 10 minutes
Servings: 2
Ingredients

- 1 egg
- 1 English muffin
- 1 turkey sausage patty
- 1 tablespoon shredded goat cheese

Directions

1. In a small skillet sprayed with non-stick cooking spray, pour egg and cook over medium-low heat. When egg appears almost cooked through, turn over with a spatula and cook an additional 30 seconds.
2. Toast English muffin.

3. Place turkey sausage patty on a plate, cover with a paper towel and cook in the microwave for 1 minute or the time recommended on the package.
4. Assemble cooked egg on English muffin (fold to fit muffin). Top with a sausage patty, then sharp goat cheese and remaining muffin half.

Nutrition: Calories: 149 Total Fat: 5.5g Cholesterol: 104mg Sodium: 368mg Total Carbohydrate: 12.8g Protein: 11.4g Calcium: 84mg Potassium: 61mg Phosphorus: 58mg

5. Denver Omelets

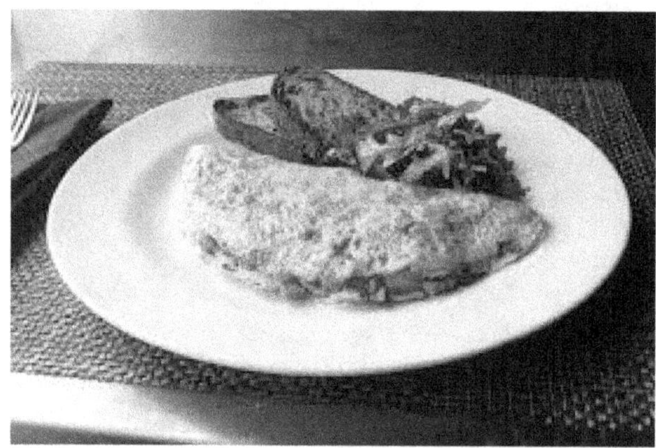

Preparation Time: 4 minutes
Cooking Time: 1 minute
Serving: 1
Ingredients

- 2 tablespoons almond butter
- ¼ cup onion, chopped
- ¼ cup green bell pepper, diced
- ¼ cup grape tomatoes halved
- 2 whole eggs
- ¼ cup ham, chopped

Directions

1. Take a skillet and place it over medium heat
2. Add butter and wait until the butter melts
3. Add onion and bell pepper and sauté for a few minutes
4. Take a bowl and whip eggs
5. Add the remaining ingredients and stir
6. Add sautéed onion and pepper, stir
7. Microwave the egg mix for 1 minute
8. Serve hot!

Nutrition: Calories: 605 Fat: 46g Carbohydrates: 6g Protein: 39g

6. Garlic-Mint Scrambled Eggs

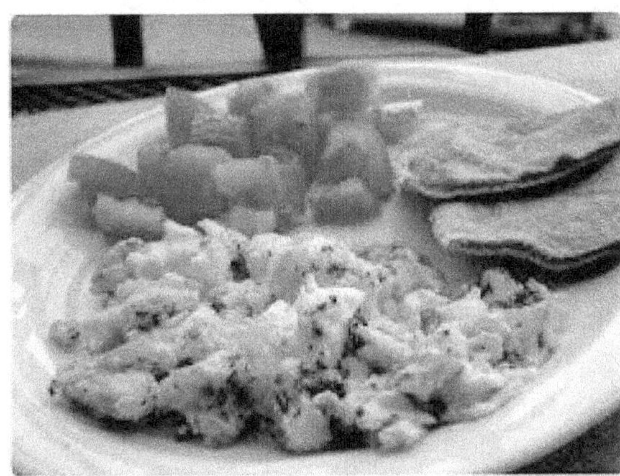

Preparation Time: 10 minutes
Cooking Time: 5 minutes
Servings: 2
Ingredients

- 4 large eggs
- ¼ cup soy milk
- 1 clove garlic, minced
- ¼ cup chopped fresh mint
- Pepper to taste

- 1 tablespoon olive oil
- ½ teaspoons freshly grated Parmesan cheese

Directions

1. Whisk together eggs, soy milk, and minced garlic until smooth; add mint and season to taste with pepper.
2. Heat olive oil in a non-stick skillet over medium heat. Pour in the egg mixture and cook to the desired degree of doneness, stirring constantly.

Nutrition: Calories: 238 Sodium: 192mg Protein:15.2g Potassium: 229mg Phosphorus: 107mg

7. Healthy Fruit Smoothie

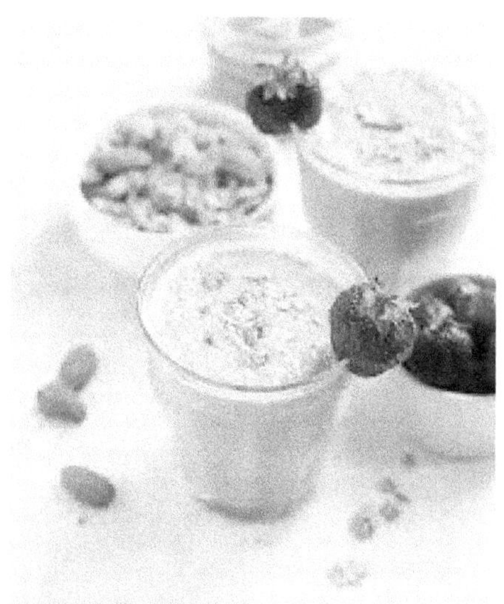

Preparation Time: 10 minutes
Cooking Time: 00 minutes
Servings: 2
Ingredients

- 1/3 cup fresh blueberries

- 1/3 cup fresh raspberries
- 4 large fresh strawberries, hulled
- 1/3 cup water
- 2/3 cup almond milk
- 2 tablespoons honey

Directions

1. Place the blueberries, raspberries, strawberries, water, milk, and honey into a blender. Cover, and puree until smooth. Pour into glasses to serve.

Nutrition: Calories: 284 Sodium: 15mg Protein: 2.6g Calcium: 26mg Potassium: 326mg Phosphorus: 117mg

8. Zucchini with Egg

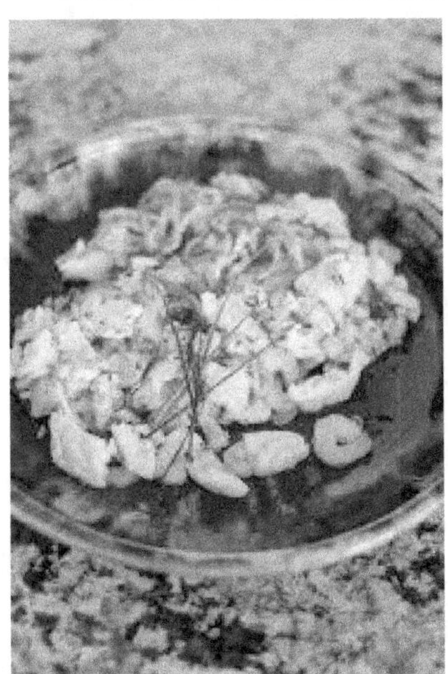

Preparation Time: 5 minutes
Cooking Time: 15 minutes
Servings: 2

Ingredients

- ½ tablespoons olive oil
- 2 large zucchini, cut into large chunks
- Ground black pepper to taste
- 2 large egg whites

Directions

1. Heat olive oil in a skillet over medium-high heat; sauté zucchini until tender, about 10 minutes. Season zucchini with black pepper.
2. Beat egg whites with a fork in a bowl; Pour eggs over zucchini; cook and stir until eggs are scrambled and no longer runny, about 5 minutes. Season zucchini and eggs with black pepper. Serve and enjoy.

Nutrition: Calories: 99 Total Sodium: 66mg Protein: 7.5g Potassium: 91mg Phosphorus: 71mg

9. Green Slime Smoothie

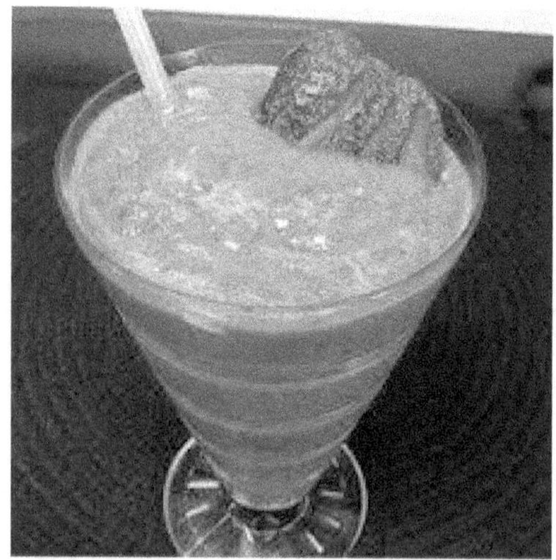

Preparation Time: 5 minutes

Cooking Time: 00 minutes
Servings: 2
Ingredients

- 1 cup kale
- 1 cup blueberries
- 1 tablespoon honey
- ¼ cup ice

Directions

1. Combine the kale, blueberries, honey, and ice in a blender. Blend until smooth.
2. Serve immediately.

Nutrition: Calories: 90 Sodium: 15mg Protein: 1.6g Calcium: 46mg Potassium: 226mg Phosphorus: 171mg

10.   Baked Omelets Roll

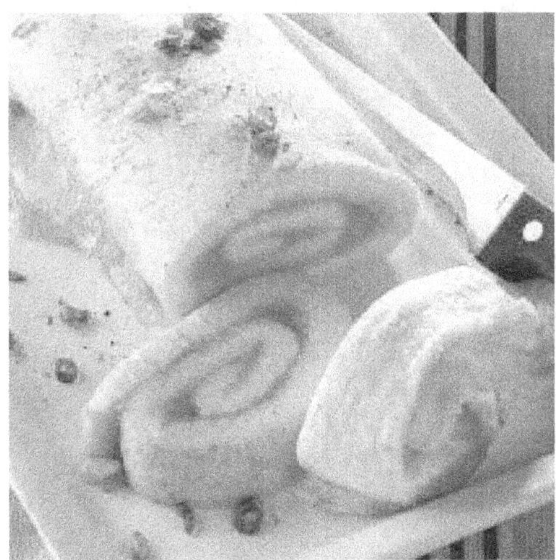

Preparation Time: 5 minutes
Cooking Time: 20 minutes
Servings: 2

Ingredients

- 2 egg whites
- ¼ cup soy milk
- 1/8 cup white flour
- 1/8 teaspoon ground black pepper
- ¼ cup shredded Cheddar cheese

Directions

1. Preheat oven to 450 degrees F. Lightly grease a 9x13-inch baking pan.
2. In a blender, combine egg whites, soy milk, almond flour, and pepper; cover and process until smooth. Pour into prepared baking pan.
3. Bake in the preheated oven until set, about 20 minutes. Sprinkle with cheese.
4. Carefully loosen edges of omelet from pan. Starting from the short edge of the pan, carefully roll up omelet. Place omelet seam side down on a serving plate and cut into 4 equal-sized pieces

Nutrition: Calories: 177 Total Fat: 13.1g Saturated Fat: 4.7g Sodium: 165mg Total Carbohydrate: 4g Protein. 11.6g Calcium: 148mg Potassium: 111mg Phosphorus: 91mg

11.   Fresh Peaches Omelets

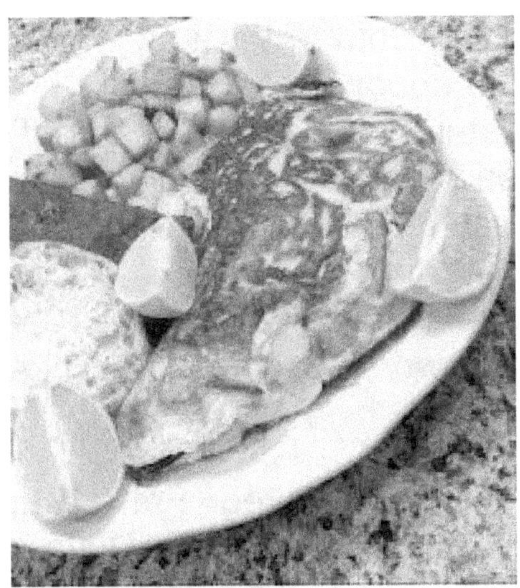

Preparation Time: 10 minutes
Cooking Time: 10 minutes
Servings: 2
Ingredients

- 1 egg white
- 1-1/2 tablespoons honey
- 1-1/2 tablespoons all-purpose flour
- 1/8 teaspoon baking powder
- 1 tablespoon almond milk
- ½ tablespoon lemon juice
- ½ teaspoon olive oil
- 1 large peach – peeled, cored and thinly sliced
- 1/8 teaspoon ground cinnamon

Directions

1. Preheat the oven to 350 degrees F.
2. In a medium bowl, whip egg white with an electric mixer until foamy. Sprinkle in honey, continuing to whip until stiff peaks form. In a separate bowl, stir together the flour, baking powder, and pepper. Mix in the almond milk and

lemon juice until well blended, then fold in the egg whites using a rubber spatula or wooden spoon.

3. Heat the olive oil in a large cast-iron (or other ovenproof) skillet over medium heat. Spread the batter evenly in the pan. Layer the thinly sliced peaches over the batter and sprinkle with cinnamon.
4. Place the skillet in the oven, and bake for 10 minutes, or until the peaches are golden brown and glazed looking. Cut into wedges to serve.

Nutrition: Calories: 113 Total Fat: 3.3g Saturated Fat: 1.8g Cholesterol: 0mg Sodium: 19mg Total Carbohydrate: 19.5g Dietary Fiber: 1.6g Total Sugars: 16.1g Protein: 3.1g Calcium: 19mg Potassium: 235mg Phosphorus: 131 mg

12.   Caramelized French Toast

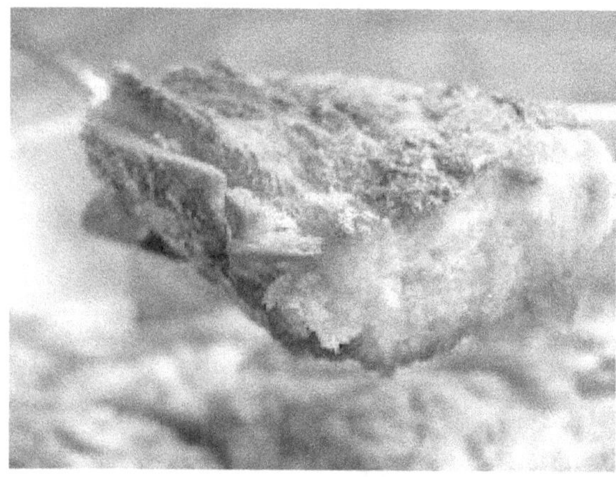

Preparation Time: 10 minutes
Cooking Time: 10 minutes
Servings: 2
Ingredients

- 1 tablespoon olive oil, divided
- 1 egg
- 1/8 cup almond milk

- 2 slices white bread
- ¼ cup brown sugar
- ¼ cup water

Directions

1. Heat ½ tablespoon of olive oil in a frying pan or skillet over medium-high heat.
2. Beat together egg, and almond milk. Dip bread one at a time into the egg mixture and fry until light brown and egg are cooked.
3. After all bread slices have been cooked and removed from the pan, add brown sugar to the pan. Stir until melted and sticky. Add water and stir. Place French toast in caramel sauce. Turn to coat, then remove from pan. Serve.

NutritionCalories: 219 Total Fat: 13.1g Saturated Fat: 4.9g Cholesterol: 82mg Sodium: 100mg
Total Carbohydrate: 23.3g Total Sugars: 18.7g Protein: 3.8g
Calcium: 44mg Potassium: 102mg Phosphorus: 81mg

13. Egg Sandwich

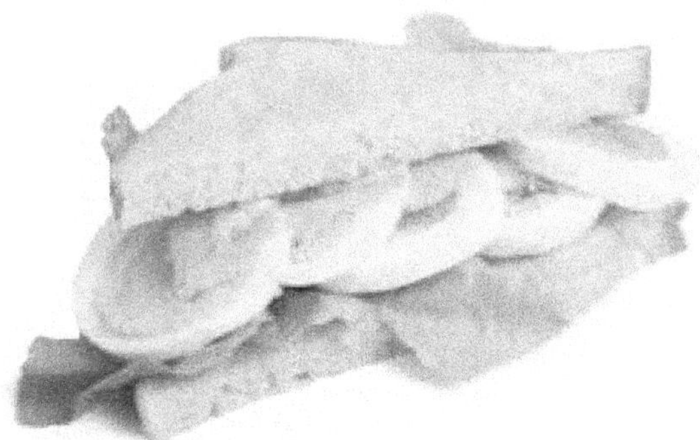

Preparation Time: 10 minutes
Cooking Time: 10 minutes
Servings: 2

Ingredients

- 2 egg whites
- 2 tablespoons almond milk
- 4 slices white bread
- Pepper to taste (optional)
- 2 slice American cheese

Directions

1. Crack the egg into a microwave-safe cereal bowl and whisk in the milk. Season with pepper. Cook in the microwave on 100% power for 1 to 2 minutes, or until cooked through. While the egg is cooking, toast the bread. Use a spoon to remove the cooked egg from the bowl and set it on one piece of toast. Top with a slice of cheese and the other piece of toast. Cook in the microwave until cheese is melted about 15 seconds

Nutrition: Calories:169 Total Fat: 9.5g Saturated Fat: 6.4g Cholesterol: 17mg Sodium: 424mg Total Carbohydrate: 11.8g Total Sugars: 3.1g Protein: 9.2g Calcium: 152mg Potassium: 172mg Phosphorus: 100mg

14. Breakfast Tacos

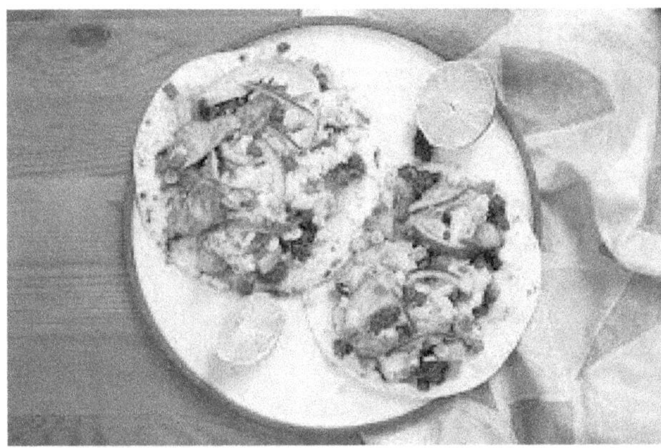

Preparation Time: 10 minutes
Cooking Time: 10 minutes
Servings: 4

Ingredients

- 1 teaspoon olive oil
- ½ sweet onion, chopped
- ½ red bell pepper, chopped
- ½ teaspoon minced garlic
- 4 eggs, beaten
- ½ teaspoon ground cumin
- Pinch red pepper flakes
- 4 tortillas
- ¼ cup tomato salsa

Directions

1. Heat the oil in a large skillet in a medium heat only.
2. Add the onion, bell pepper, and garlic, and sauté until softened, about 5 minutes.
3. Add the eggs, cumin, and red pepper flakes, and scramble the eggs with the vegetables until cooked through and fluffy.

4. Spoon one-fourth of the egg mixture into the center of each tortilla, and top each with 1 tablespoon of salsa.
5. Serve immediately.

Nutrition: Calories: 331 kcal Total Fat: 11 g Sodium: 35 mg Total Carbs: 52 g Protein: 6 g

15.   Fruit and Cheese Breakfast Wrap

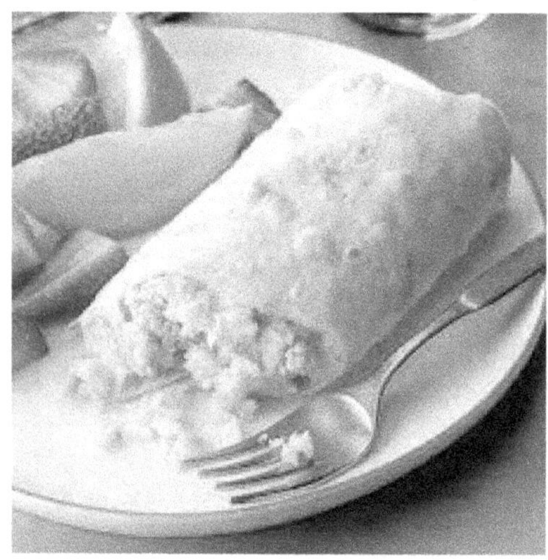

Preparation Time: 10 minutes
Cooking Time: 0 minutes
Servings: 2
Ingredients

- Flour tortillas – 2 (6-inch)
- Plain cream cheese – 2 tbsp.
- Apple – 1, peeled, cored, and sliced thinly
- Honey – 1 tbsp.

Directions

1. Lay both tortillas on a clean work surface and spread 1 tbsp. of cream cheese onto each tortilla, leaving about ½

inch around the edges.

2. Arrange the apple slices on the cream cheese, just off the center of the tortilla on the side closest to you, leaving about 1 ½ inch on each side and 2 inches on the bottom.
3. Drizzle the apples lightly with honey.
4. Fold the left and right edges of the tortillas into the center, laying the edge over the apples.
5. Taking the tortilla edge closest to you, fold it over the fruit and the side pieces.
6. Roll the tortilla away from you, creating a snug wrap.
7. Repeat with the second tortilla.

Nutrition: Calories: 188 kcal Total Fat: 6 g Sodium: 177 mg Total Carbs: 33 g Protein: 4 g

16. Mozzarella Cheese Omelet

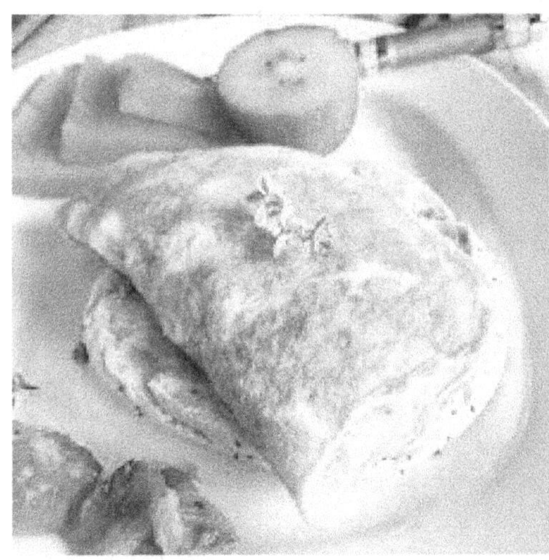

Preparation time: 10 minutes
Cooking time: 5 minutes
Servings: 1
Ingredients

- 4 eggs, beaten

- 1/4 cup mozzarella cheese, shredded
- 4 tomato slices
- 1/4 tablespoon Italian seasoning
- 1/4 tablespoon dried oregano
- Pepper
- Salt

Directions

1. In a small bowl, whisk eggs with salt.
2. Spray the pan with cooking spray and heat over medium heat.
3. Pour egg mixture into the pan and cook over medium heat.
4. Once eggs are set, then sprinkle oregano and Italian seasoning on top.
5. Arrange tomato slices on top of the omelet and sprinkle with shredded cheese.
6. Cook omelet for 1 minute.
7. Serve and enjoy.

Nutrition: Calories: 285 Fat: 19g Carbohydrates: 4g Sugar: 3g Protein: 25g Cholesterol: 655mg

17. Sun-Dried Tomato Frittata

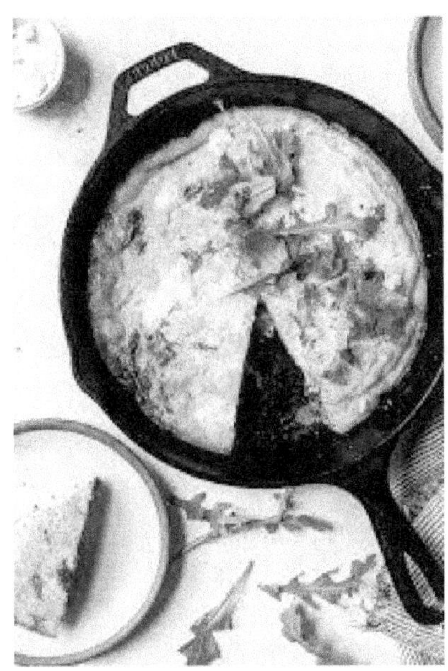

Preparation time: 10 minutes
Cooking time: 20 minutes
Servings: 8
Ingredients

- 12 eggs
- 1/2 tablespoon dried basil
- 1/4 cup parmesan cheese, grated
- 2 cups baby spinach, shredded
- 1/4 cup sun-dried tomatoes, sliced
- Pepper
- Salt

Directions

1. Preheat the oven to 425°F. In a large bowl, whisk eggs with pepper and salt.
2. Add remaining ingredients and stir to combine. Spray oven-safe pan with cooking spray.
3. Pour egg mixture into the pan and bake for 20 minutes.

4. Slice and serve.

Nutrition: Calories: 115 Fat: 7g Carbohydrates: 1g Sugar: 1g
Protein: 10g Cholesterol: 250mg

18.   Italian Breakfast Frittata

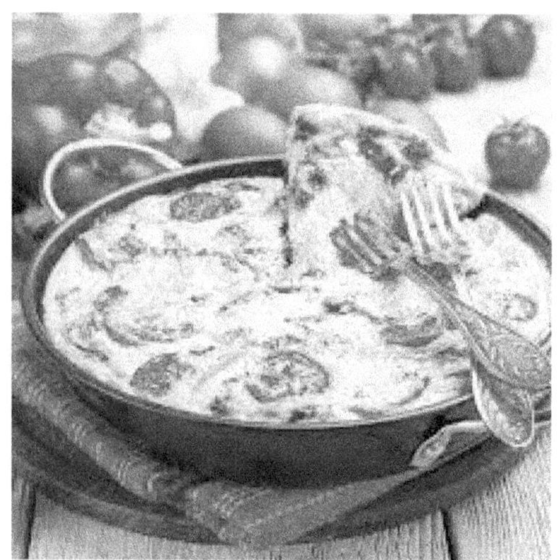

Preparation time: 10 minutes
Cooking time: 45 minutes
Servings: 4
Ingredients

- 2 cups egg whites
- 1/2 cup mozzarella cheese, shredded
- 1 cup cottage cheese, crumbled
- 1/4 cup fresh basil, sliced
- 1/2 cup roasted red peppers, sliced
- Pepper
- Salt

Directions

1. Preheat the oven to 375ºF.

2. Add all ingredients into the large bowl and whisk well to combine.
3. Pour frittata mixture into the baking dish and bake for 45 minutes.
4. Slice and serve.

Nutrition: Calories: 131 Fat: 2g Carbohydrates: 5g Sugar: 2g Protein: 22g Cholesterol: 6mg

19.   Baked Cheese and Sausage Omelet

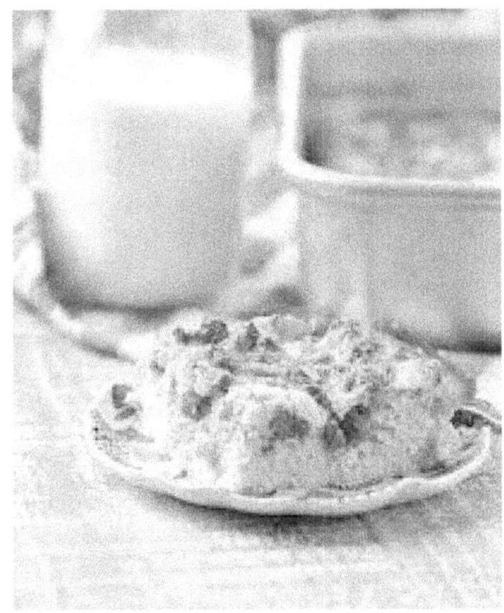

Preparation time: 10 minutes
Cooking time: 45 minutes
Servings: 8
Ingredients

- 16 eggs
- 2 cups cheddar cheese, shredded
- 1/2 cup salsa
- 1lb ground sausage
- 1 1/2 cups coconut milk
- Pepper

- Salt

Directions

1. Preheat the oven to 350ºF.
2. Add the sausage to a pan and cook until browned. Drain excess fat.
3. In a large bowl, whisk eggs and milk. Stir in cheese, cooked sausage, and salsa.
4. Pour omelet mixture into the baking dish and bake for 45 minutes.
5. Serve and enjoy.

Nutrition: Calories: 360 Fat: 24g Carbohydrates: 4g Sugar: 3g Protein: 28g Cholesterol: 400mg

20.   Greek Egg Scrambled

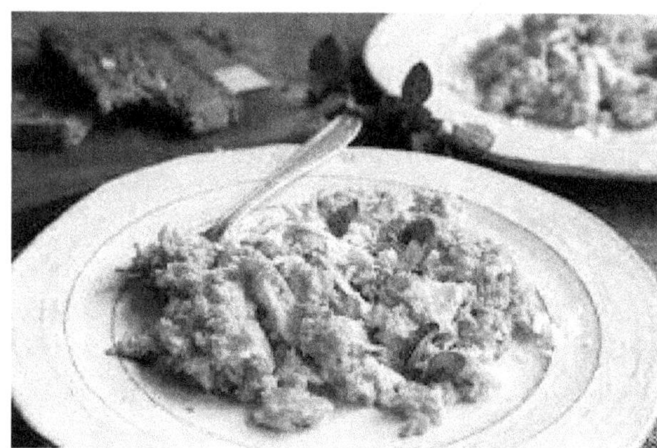

Preparation time: 10 minutes
Cooking time: 10 minutes
Servings: 2
Ingredients

- 4 eggs
- 1/2 cup grape tomatoes, sliced

- 2 tablespoon green onions, sliced
- 1 bell pepper, diced
- 1 tablespoon olive oil
- 1/4 tablespoon dried oregano
- 1/2 tablespoon capers
- 3 olives, sliced
- Pepper
- Salt

Directions

1. Heat oil in a pan over medium heat.
2. Add green onions and bell pepper and cook until pepper is softened.
3. Add tomatoes, capers, and olives and cook for 1 minute.
4. Add eggs and stir until eggs are cooked. Season it with oregano, pepper, and salt.
5. Serve and enjoy.

Nutrition: Calories: 230 Fat: 17g Carbohydrates: 8g Sugar: 5g Protein: 12g Cholesterol: 325mg

21.   Apple-Cinnamon Drink

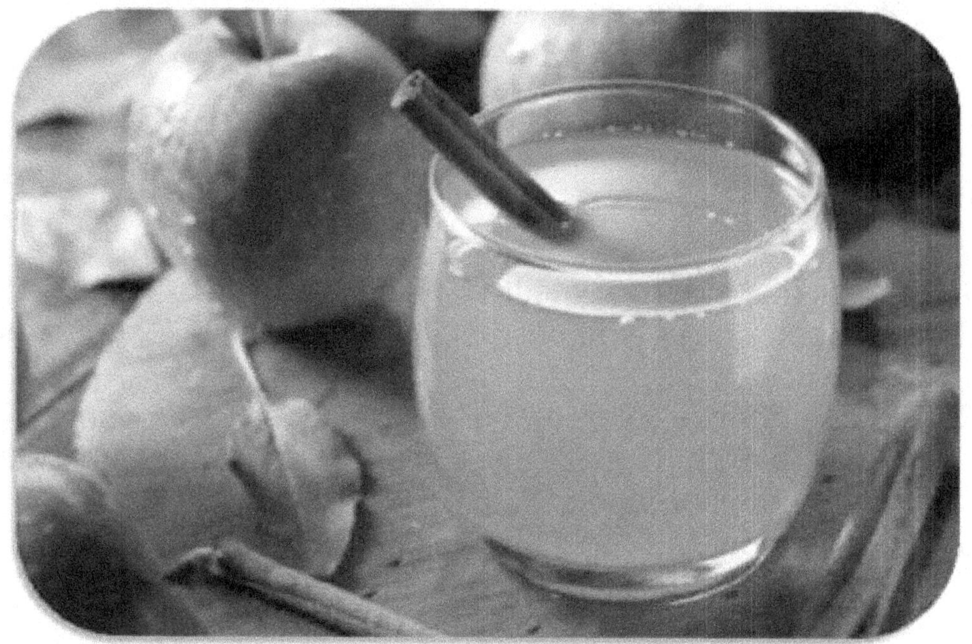

Preparation time: 10 minutes
Cooking time: 5 minutes
Servings: 8
Ingredients

- 10 cups water
- 1 medium apple, sliced
- 2 cinnamon sticks
- 2 teaspoons ground cinnamon

Direction:

1. Add apple slices, water, and cinnamon to a blender.

2. Pour this mixture, along with cinnamon stick, into a suitable cooking pot and cook for 5 minutes.
3. Strain the apple-cinnamon water and allow it to cool.
4. Serve.

Nutrition: Calories: 4 Protein: 0 g Carbohydrates: 1 g Fat: 0 g Cholesterol: 0 mg Sodium: 7 mg Potassium: 10 mg

22. Blackberry-Sage Drink

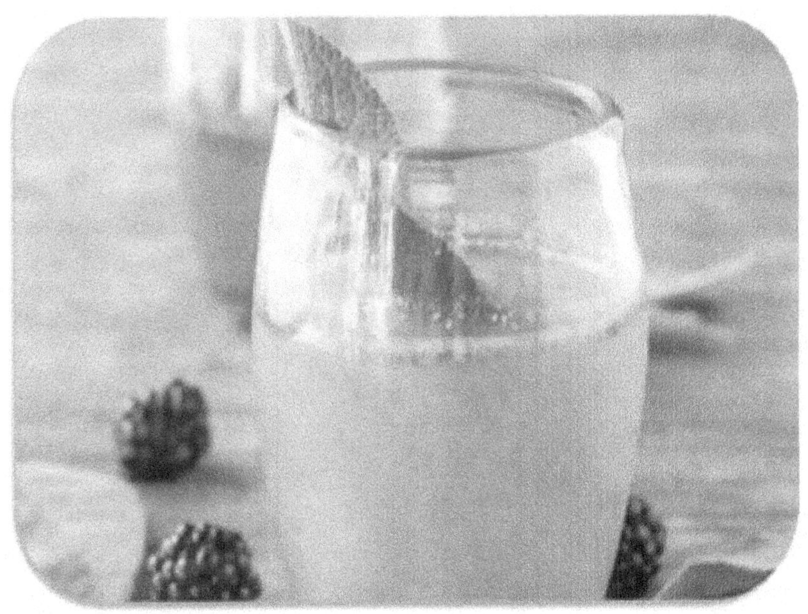

Preparation time: 10 minutes
Cooking time: 0 minutes
Servings: 8
Ingredients

- 1 cup fresh blackberries
- 4 sage leaves
- 10 cups water

Direction:

1. Add blackberries, sage leave, and 10 cups water to a
   blender.
2. Blend well, then strain and refrigerate to chill.
3. Serve.

Nutrition: Calories: 7 Protein: 0 g Carbohydrates: 2 g Fat: 0 g
Cholesterol: 0 mg Sodium: 7 mg Potassium: 26 mg

23. Beet Juice Blend

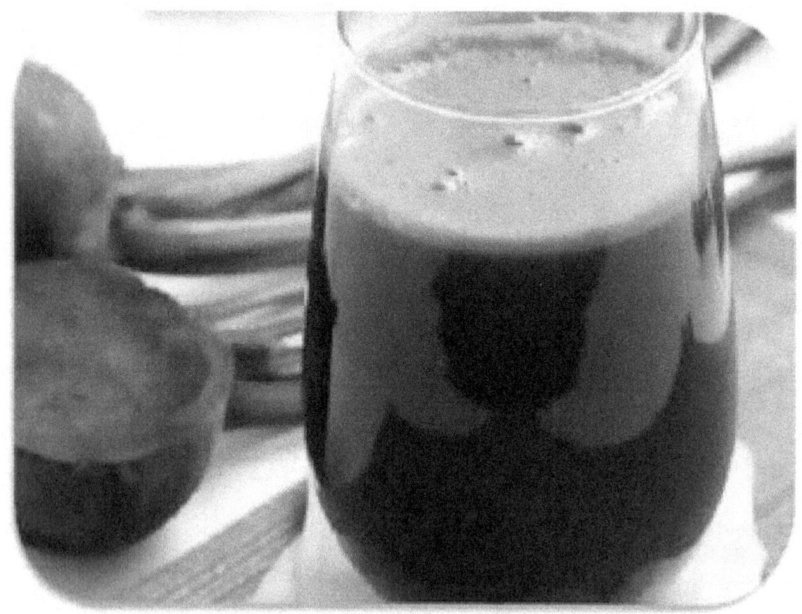

Preparation time: 10 minutes
Cooking time: 0 minutes
Servings: 2
Ingredients

- ½ medium apple
- ½ medium beet
- 1 medium fresh carrot
- 1 celery stalk

- ¼ cup parsley

Direction:

1. Pass apple, beet, celery, parsley, and carrot through a juicer.
2. Divide this juice into two serving glasses, then refrigerate to chill.
3. Serve.

Nutrition: Calories: 186 Protein: 23 g Carbohydrates: 19 g Fat: 2 g Cholesterol: 41 mg Sodium: 62 mg Potassium: 282 mg

24. Caramel Protein Latte

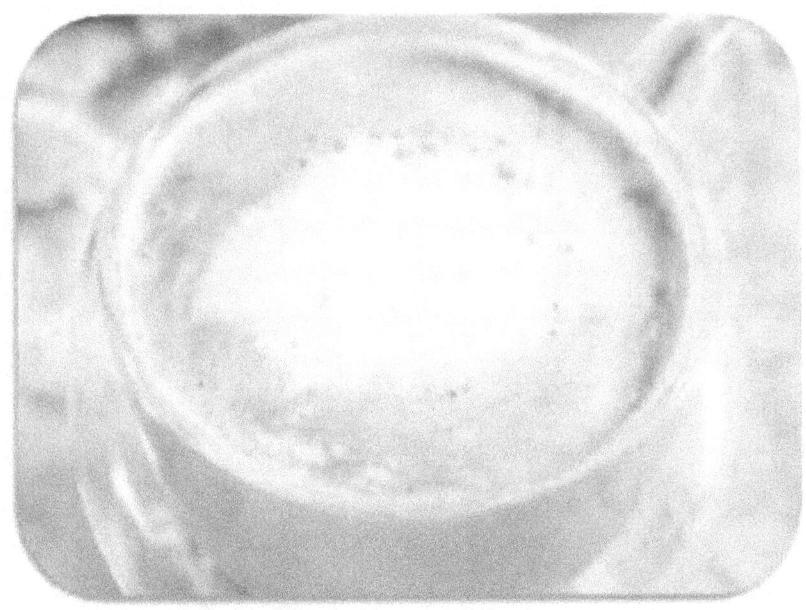

Preparation time: 10 minutes
Cooking time: 0 minutes
Servings: 2
Ingredients

- 1 scoop whey protein powder
- 2 ounces water
- 6 ounces hot coffee
- 2 tablespoons caramel syrup

Direction:

1. Mix 1 scoop of protein powder with 2 ounces of water in a mug.
2. Pour in 6 ounces of hot coffee, then mix well.
3. Stir in sugar-free syrup and serve.

Nutrition: Calories: 72 Protein: 17 g Carbohydrates: 1 g Fat: 0 g Cholesterol: 0 mg Sodium: 55 mg Potassium: 214 mg

25. Cinnamon Smoothie

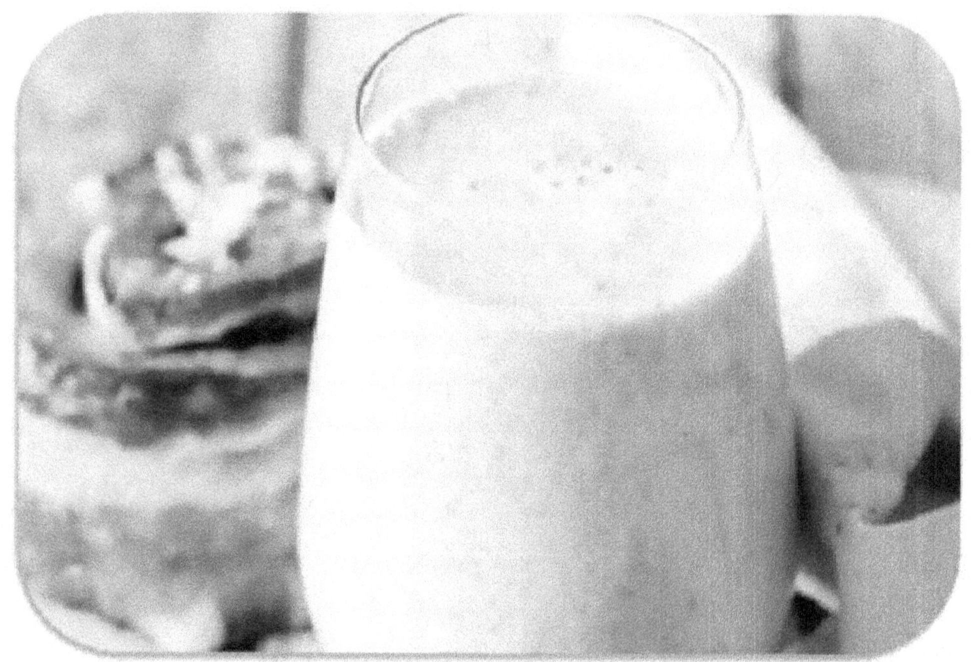

Preparation time: 10 minutes

Cooking time: 0 minutes
Servings: 2
Ingredients

- ½ teaspoon ground cinnamon
- 1 tablespoon sugar
- 1/8 teaspoon vanilla extract
- 8 ounces egg white
- 3 tablespoons whipped topping

Direction:

1. Mix cinnamon, sugar, 2 ounces egg whites, and vanilla in a mixer.
2. Serve with whipped topping.
3. Enjoy.

Nutrition: Calories: 207 Protein: 28 g Carbohydrates: 17 g Fat: 3 g Cholesterol: 0 mg Sodium: 428 mg Potassium: 427 mg

26.　Citrus Shake

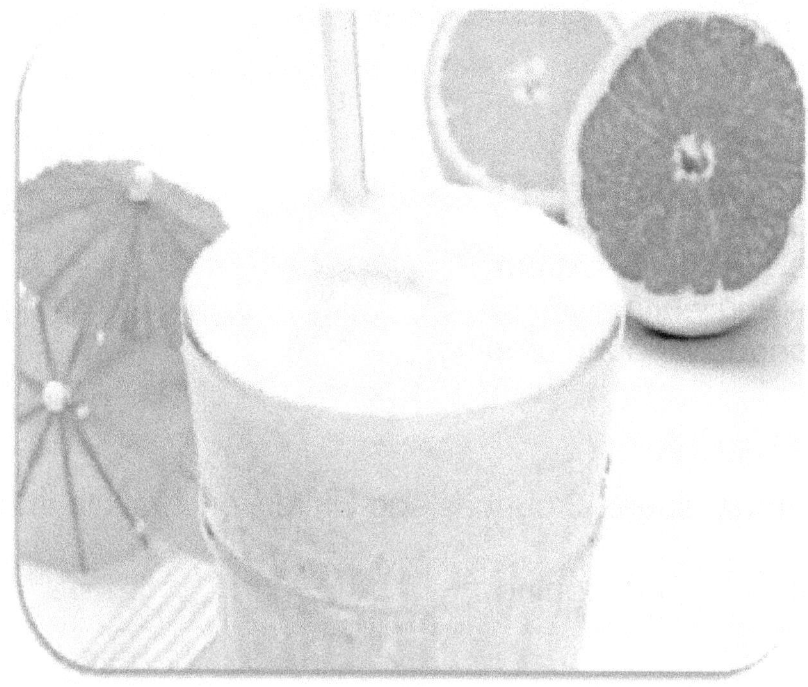

Preparation time: 10 minutes
Cooking time: 0 minutes
Servings: 2
Ingredients

- ½ cup pineapple juice
- ½ cup almond milk
- 1 cup orange sherbet
- ½ cup egg

Direction:

1. Pour almond milk, sherbet, pineapple juice, and egg into a blender.
2. Blend well for 30 seconds, then refrigerate to chill.
3. Serve.

Nutrition: Calories: 190 Protein: 7 g Carbohydrates: 36 g Fat: 2 g Cholesterol: 1 mg Sodium: 192 mg
Potassium: 310 mg Phosphorus: 83 mg Calcium: 205 mg Fiber: 1.3 g

27. Pineapple Protein Smoothie

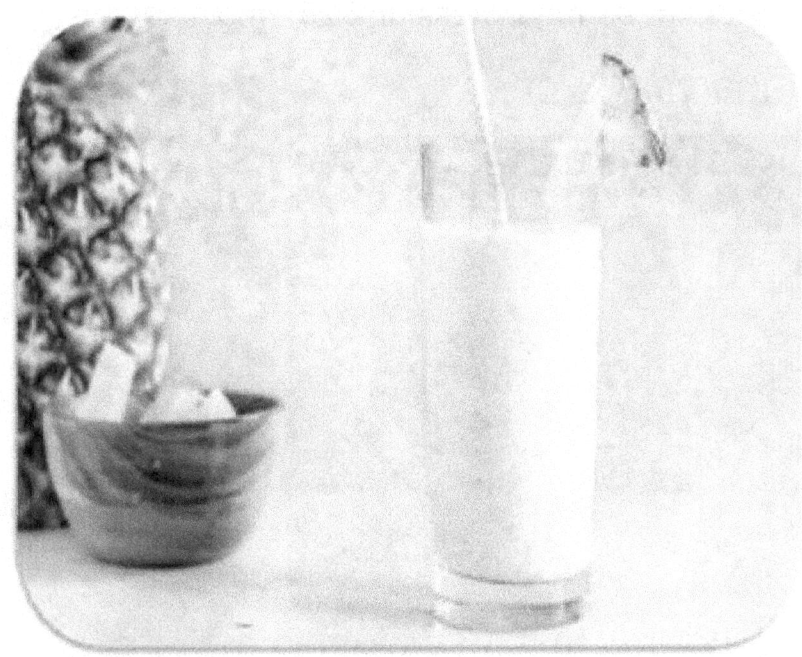

Preparation time: 10 minutes
Cooking time: 0 minutes
Servings: 2
Ingredients

- ¾ cup pineapple sherbet
- 1 scoop vanilla protein powder
- ½ cup water
- 2 ice cubes

Direction:

1. Add pineapple sherbet, water, protein powder, and ice cubes to a blender.
2. Blend the pineapple smoothie for 45 seconds.
3. Serve.

Nutrition: Calories: 268 Protein: 18 g Carbohydrates: 40 g Fat: 4 g Cholesterol: 36 mg Sodium: 93 mg Potassium: 237 mg

28.   Hazelnut Cinnamon Coffee

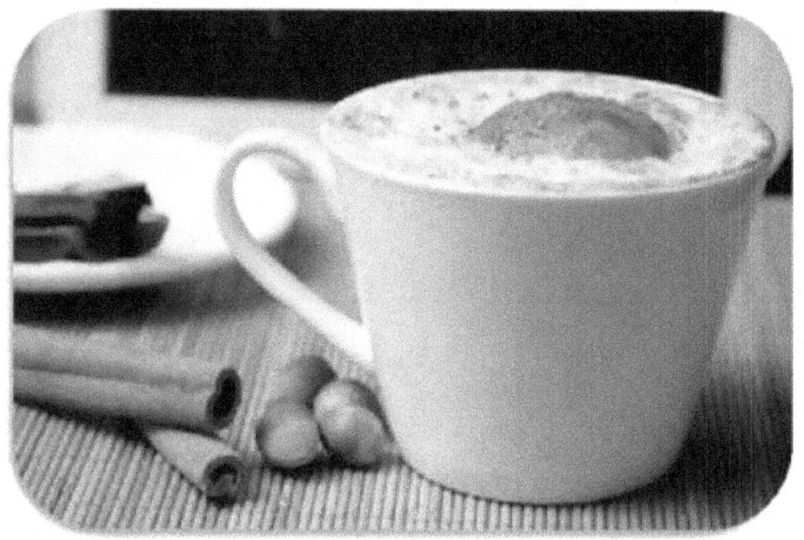

Preparation time: 10 minutes
Cooking time: 0 minutes
Servings: 4
Ingredients

- 4 cups brewed coffee
- 8 teaspoons hazelnut syrup
- 4 tablespoons milk
- 4 cinnamon sticks

Direction:

1. Start by brewing coffee in a coffee maker, then divide it into the small cups.
2. Add 2 teaspoons hazelnut syrup, 1 tablespoon milk, and 2 cinnamon sticks to each mug.
3. Serve.

Nutrition: Calories: 13 Protein: 1 g Carbohydrates: 1 g Fat: 0 g Cholesterol: 1 mg Sodium: 13 mg Potassium: 139 mg

29.   Protein Piña Colada

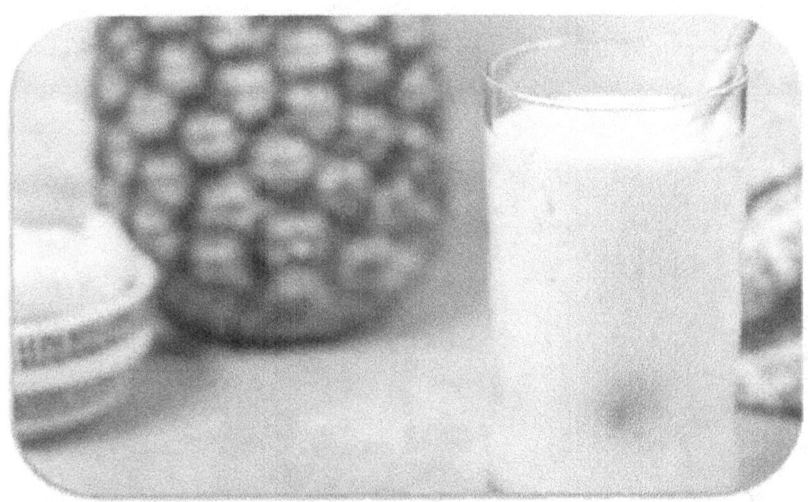

Preparation time: 10 minutes
Cooking time: 0 minutes
Servings: 1
Ingredients

- 6 ounces pineapple juice
- 1-ounce whey protein
- ½ cup crushed ice
- 1-ounce lemon-lime soda
- 2 slices fresh pineapple

Direction:

1. Add pineapple juice, protein powder, and ice to a blender jug.
2. Pour piña colada mixture into the serving glasses.
3. Top the piña colada with lemon-lime soda.
4. Garnish with pineapple slices.
5. Serve.

Nutrition: Calories: 106 Protein: 12 g Carbohydrates: 14 g Fat: 0 g Cholesterol: 0 mg Sodium: 33 mg Potassium: 202 mg

30. Holiday Cider

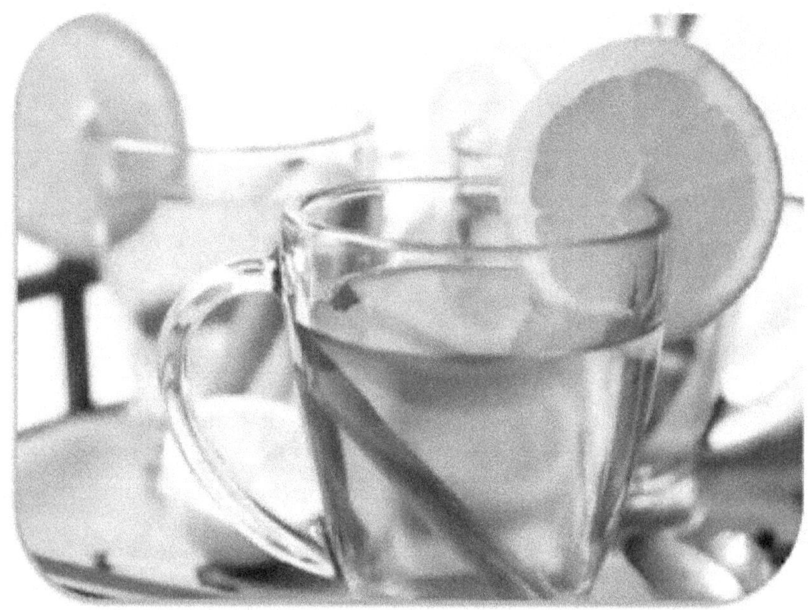

Preparation time: 10 minutes
Cooking time: 0 minutes
Servings: 8
Ingredients

- 8 cups apple cider
- 3 cinnamon sticks
- ¼ teaspoon whole cloves

- ¼ teaspoon ground allspice

Direction:

1. Add cider, cinnamon sticks, allspice, and cloves to a slow cooker.
2. Cook this apple cider mixture for 1 hour on low heat.
3. Strain and serve.

Nutrition: Calories: 68 Protein: 0 g Carbohydrates: 17 g Fat: 0 g Cholesterol: 0 mg Sodium: 34 mg Potassium: 168 mg

31.   Cinnamon and Hazelnut Coffee

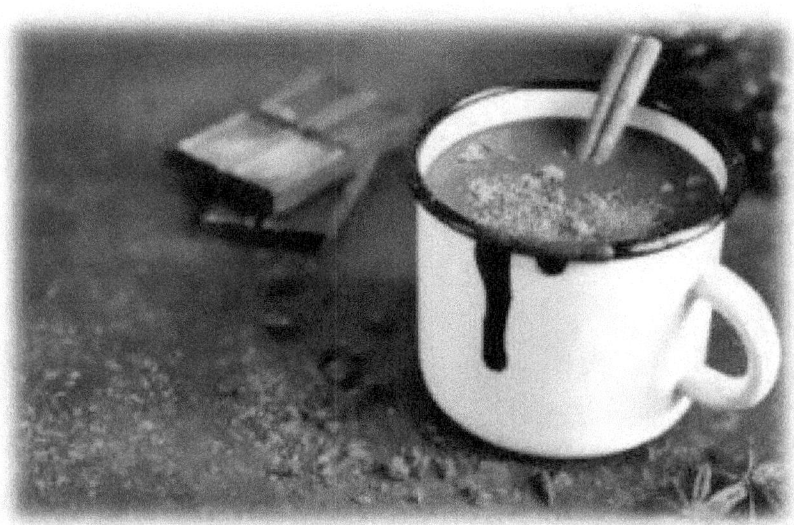

Preparation Time: 0 minutes
Cooking Time: 5 minutes
Servings – 4
Ingredients

- 4 sticks of cinnamon
- 8 teaspoons hazelnut syrup, sugar-free
- 4 tablespoons milk, low-fat

- 4 cups brewed coffee

Direction:

1. 1.Distribute brewed coffee into small cups, and then stir in 2 teaspoons of hazelnut syrup into each cup along with 1 tablespoon milk until combined.
2. 2.Garnish coffee with a stick of cinnamon and serve.

Nutrition: Calories – 13 Fat – 0 g Protein – 1 g Carbohydrates – 1 g Fiber – 0 g Sodium – 13 mg Potassium – 139 mg Phosphorus – 22 mg

32. Almond Milk

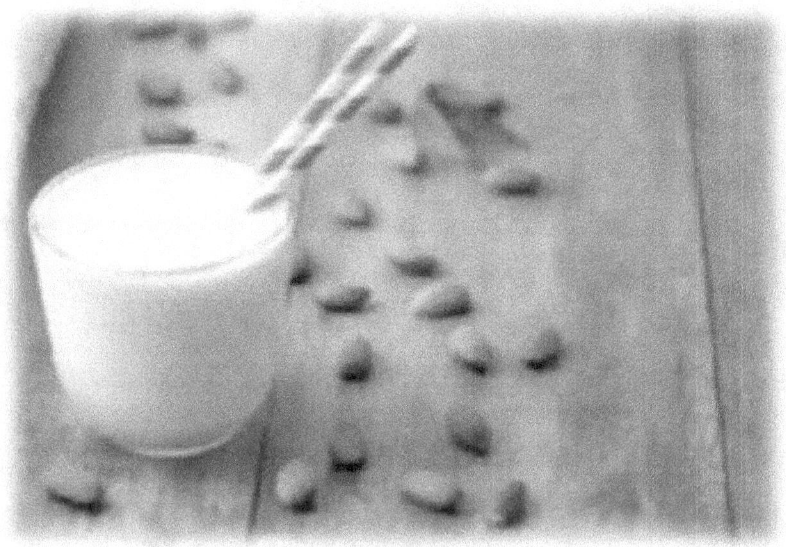

Preparation Time: 5 minutes
Cooking Time: 0 minutes
Servings – 3
Ingredients

- 1 cup almonds, soaked in warm water for 10 minutes

- 1 teaspoon vanilla extract, unsweetened
- 3 cups of filtered water

Direction:

1. 1.Drain the soaked almonds, place them into the blender, pour in water, and blend for 2 minutes until almonds are chopped.
2. 2.Strain the milk by passing it through a cheesecloth into a bowl, discard almond meal, and then stir vanilla into the milk.
3. 3.Cover the milk, refrigerate until chilled, and when ready to serve, stir it well, pour the milk evenly into the glasses and then serve.

Nutrition: Calories – 40 Fat – 3 g Protein – 1 g Carbohydrates – 2 g Fiber – 0 g Sodium – 6 mg Potassium – 180 mg Phosphorus – 40 mg

33.   Blueberry Smoothie

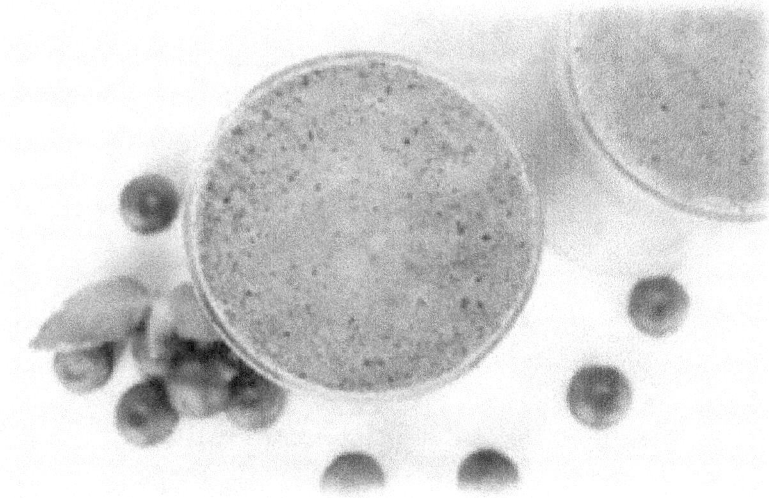

Preparation Time: 5 minutes

Cooking Time: 0 minutes
Servings – 4
Ingredients

- 1 cup frozen blueberries
- 6 tablespoons protein powder
- 8 packets of Splenda
- 14 ounces of apple juice, unsweetened
- 8 cubes of ice

Direction:

1. .Take a blender, place all the ingredients (in order) in it, and then process for 1 minute until smooth.
2. .Distribute the smoothie between four glasses and then serve.

Nutrition: Calories – 108 Fat – 0 g Protein – 9 g Carbohydrates – 18 g Fiber – 1.2 g Sodium – 27 mg Potassium – 183 mg Phosphorus – 42 mg

34.   Cucumber and Lemon-Flavored Water

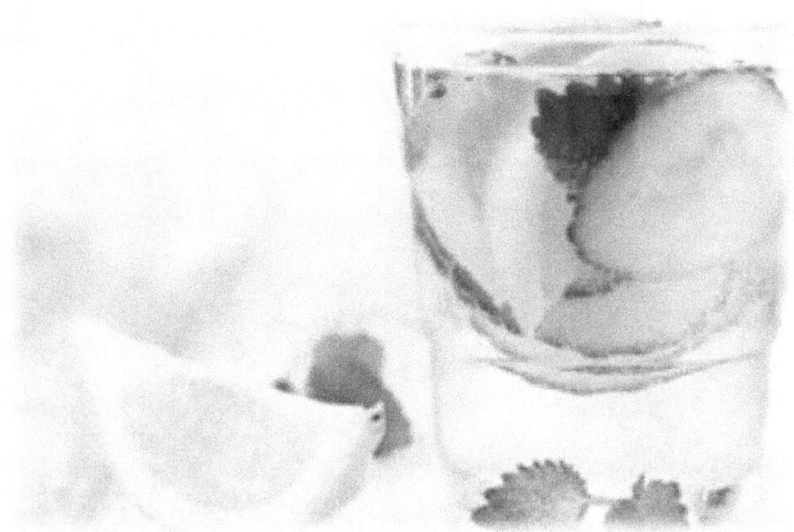

Preparation Time: 3 hours and 5 minutes
Cooking Time: 0 minutes
Servings – 10
Ingredients

- 1 lemon, deseeded, sliced
- ¼ cup fresh mint leaves, chopped
- 1 medium cucumber, sliced
- ¼ cup fresh basil leaves, chopped
- 10 cups water

Direction:

1. Take a pitcher, place all the ingredients (in order) in it, and then stir until mixed.
2. Place the pitcher in the refrigerator, chill the water for a minimum of 3 hours (or overnight), and then serve.

Nutrition: Calories – 4 Fat – 0 g Protein – 0 g Carbohydrates – 1 g Fiber – 0.4 g Sodium – 8 mg Potassium – 38 mg Phosphorus – 4 mg

35.   <u>Fruity Smoothie</u>

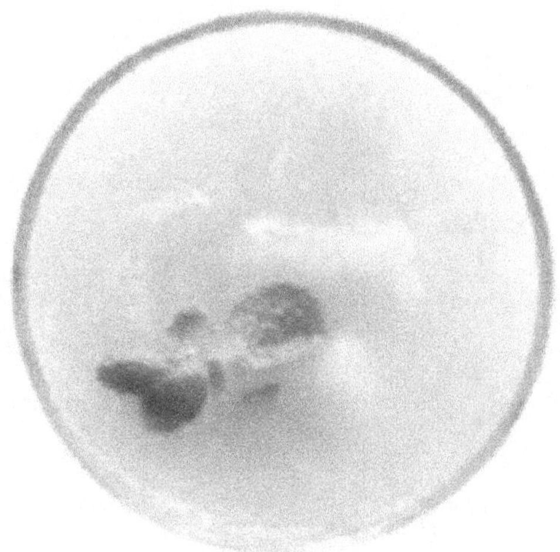

Preparation Time: 10 minutes
Cooking Time: 0 minutes
Servings – 2
Ingredients

- 2 scoops vanilla-flavored whey protein powder
- 8 ounces fruit cocktail, with juice
- 1 cup of water, cold
- 1 cup crushed ice

Direction:

1. .Take a blender, place all the ingredients (in order) in it, and then process for 30 seconds until smooth.
2. Distribute the shake between two glasses and then serve.

Nutrition: Calories – 186 Fat – 2 g Protein – 23 g Carbohydrates – 19 g Fiber – 1.1 g Sodium – 62 mg Potassium – 282 mg Phosphorus – 118 mg

36.   Hot Mulled Punch

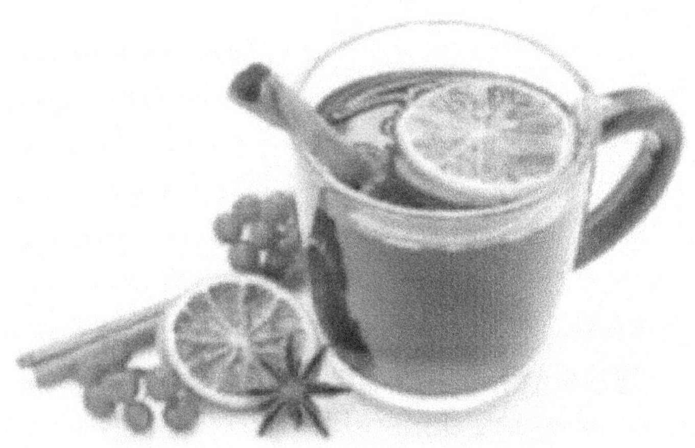

Preparation Time: 5 minutes
Cooking Time: 10 minutes
Servings – 14
Ingredients

- 4 sticks of cinnamon, broken
- ½ cup brown sugar
- 1 ½ teaspoons whole cloves
- 6 cups cranberry juice, unsweetened
- 8 cups apple juice, unsweetened

Direction:

1. .Take a large pot, place it over medium-high heat, add all the ingredients in it, and stir until mixed.
2. .Simmer the punch until hot and then serve.

Nutrition: Calories – 135 Fat – 0 g Protein – 0 g Carbohydrates – 33 g Fiber – 0.3 g Sodium – 7 mg Potassium – 267 mg Phosphorus – 25 mg

37. Lemon Smoothie

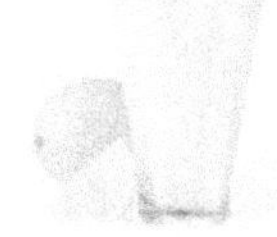

Preparation Time: 5 minutes
Cooking Time: 0 minutes
Servings – 1
Ingredients

- 4 teaspoons Splenda granulated sugar
- 3 tablespoons whipped dessert topping
- 2 teaspoons lemon juice
- 8 ounces liquid egg white, pasteurized

Direction:

1. .Take a smoothie glass, place all the ingredients in it, and stir well until whipped topping melts.
2. .Serve straight away.

Nutrition: Calories – 227 Fat – 3 g Protein – 28 g Carbohydrates – 22 g Fiber – 0 g Sodium – 428 mg Potassium – 433 mg Phosphorus – 39 mg

38. Peach Smoothie

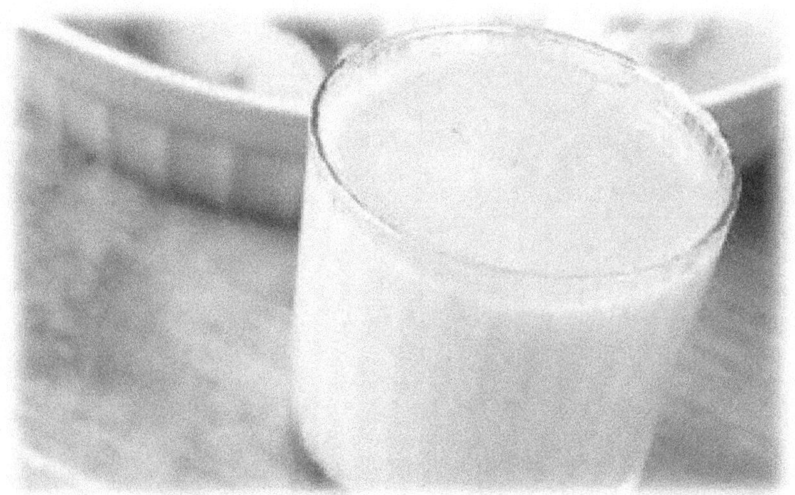

Preparation Time: 5 minutes
Cooking Time: 0 minutes
Servings – 1
Ingredients

- ¾ cup fresh peaches, diced
- 1 tablespoon Splenda granulated sugar
- 2 tablespoons powdered egg whites
- ½ cup ice

Direction:

1. .Take a blender, place peaches in it, and blend for 30 seconds until smooth.
2. .Then add remaining ingredients in a blender, pulse for 1 minute until combined, and then pour the smoothie in a glass.
3. 3.Serve straight away.

Nutrition: Calories – 132 Fat – 0 g Protein – 10 g Carbohydrates – 24 g Fiber – 1.9 g Sodium – 154 mg Potassium – 353 mg Phosphorus – 36 mg

39.   Pineapple Punch

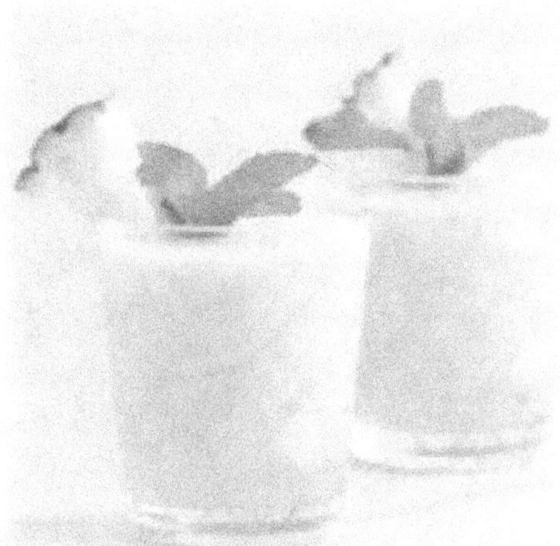

Preparation Time: 5 minutes
Cooking Time: 0 minutes
Servings – 12
Ingredients

- Pineapple slices as needed for garnishing
- 8 ounces crushed pineapple
- 4 cups pineapple juice
- 4 cups lemon-lime soda
- 4 cups of ice cubes

Direction:

1. .Take a large punch bowl, place all the ingredients in it, and stir until mixed.
2. .Pour punch into glasses, add a slice of pineapple, and then serve.

Nutrition: Calories – 120 Fat – 0 g Protein – 0 g Carbohydrates – 30 g Fiber – 0.1 g Sodium – 26 mg Potassium – 106 mg

Phosphorus – 6 mg

40.   Cinnamon Apple Chips

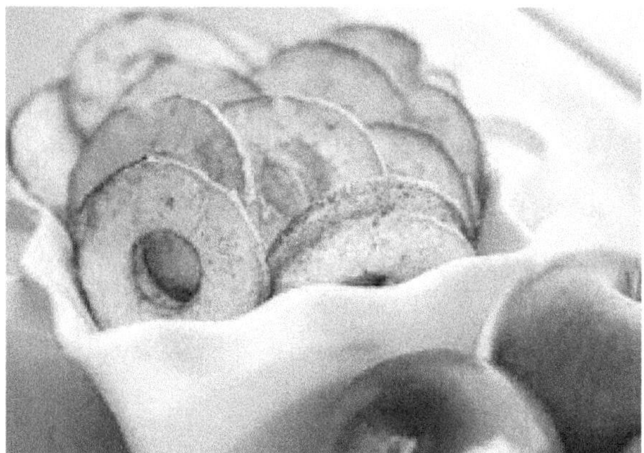

Preparation Time: 5 Minutes
Cooking Time: 2 To 3 Hours
Serving: 4
Ingredients:

- 4 apples
- 1 teaspoon ground cinnamon

Direction:

1. Preheat the oven to 200°F. Line a baking sheet with parchment paper.
2. Core the apples and cut into 1/8-inch slices.
3. In a medium bowl, toss the apple slices with the cinnamon. Spread the apples in a single layer on the prepared baking sheet.
4. Cook for 2 to 3 hours, until the apples are dry. They will still be soft while hot, but will crisp once completely cooled. Store in an airtight container for up to four days.

Cooking tip: If you don't have parchment paper, use cooking spray to prevent sticking.

NutritionPer Serving Calories: 96; Total Fat: 0g; Saturated Fat: 0g; Cholesterol: 0mg; Carbohydrates: 26g; Fiber: 5g; Protein: 1g; Phosphorus: 0mg; Potassium: 198mg; Sodium: 2mg

41. Savory Collard Chips

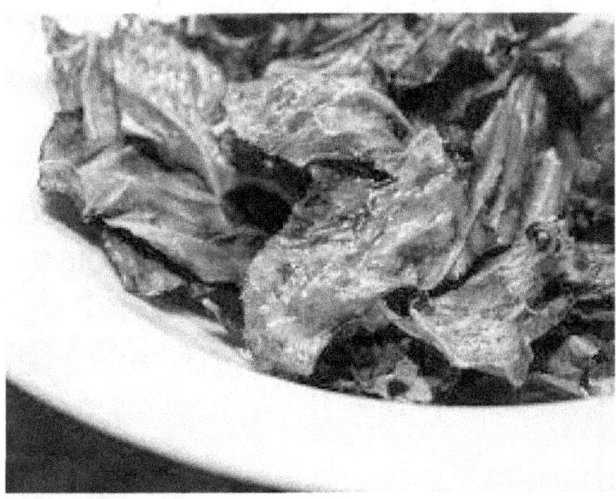

Preparation Time: 5 Minutes
Cooking Time: 20 Minutes
Serving: 4
Ingredients:

- 1 bunch collard greens
- 1 teaspoon extra-virgin olive oil
- Juice of ½ lemon
- ½ teaspoon garlic powder
- ¼ teaspoon freshly ground black pepper

Direction:

1. Preheat the oven to 350°F. Line a baking sheet with parchment paper.

2. Cut the collards into 2-by-2-inch squares and pat dry with paper towels. In a large bowl, toss the greens with the olive oil, lemon juice, garlic powder, and pepper. Use your hands to mix well, massaging the dressing into the greens until evenly coated.
3. Arrange the collards in a single layer on the baking sheet, and cook for 8 minutes. Flip the pieces and cook for an additional 8 minutes, until crisp. Remove from the oven, let cool, and store in an airtight container in a cool location for up to three days.

Substitution tip: If you prefer, use fresh garlic instead of dried. Mince 2 or 3 cloves, toss with the collards, and proceed as directed.
NutritionPer Serving Calories: 24; Total Fat: 1g; Saturated Fat: 0g; Cholesterol: 0mg; Carbohydrates: 3g; Fiber: 1g; Protein: 1g; Phosphorus: 6mg; Potassium: 72mg; Sodium: 8mg

42.   Roasted Red Pepper Hummus

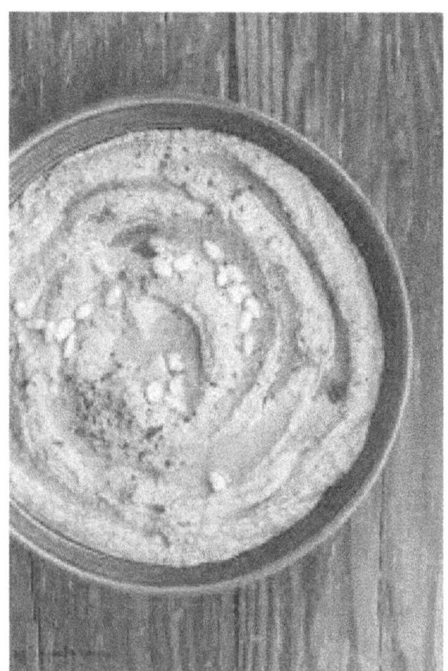

Preparation Time: 10 Minutes

Cooking Time: 10 Minutes
Serving: 8
Ingredients:

- 1 red bell pepper
- 1 (15-ounce) can chickpeas, drained and rinsed
- Juice of 1 lemon
- 2 tablespoons tahini
- 2 garlic cloves
- 2 tablespoons extra-virgin olive oil

Direction:

1. Move an oven rack to the highest position. Heat the broiler to high.
2. Core the pepper and cut it into three or four large pieces. Arrange them on a baking sheet, skin-side up.
3. Broil the peppers for 5 to 10 minutes, until the skins are charred. Remove from the oven and transfer the peppers to a small bowl. Cover with plastic wrap and let them steam for 10 to 15 minutes, until cool enough to handle.
4. Peel the charred skin off the peppers, and place the peppers in a blender.
5. Add the chickpeas, lemon juice, tahini, garlic, and olive oil. Process until smooth, adding up to 1 tablespoon of water to adjust consistency as desired.

Substitution tip: This hummus can also be made without the red pepper if desired. To do this, simply follow Step 5. This will cut the potassium to 59mg per serving.

NutritionPer Serving Calories: 103; Total Fat: 6g; Saturated Fat: 1g; Cholesterol: 0mg; Carbohydrates: 10g; Fiber: 3g; Protein: 3g; Phosphorus: 58mg; Potassium: 91mg; Sodium: 72mg

43.　Thai-Style Eggplant Dip

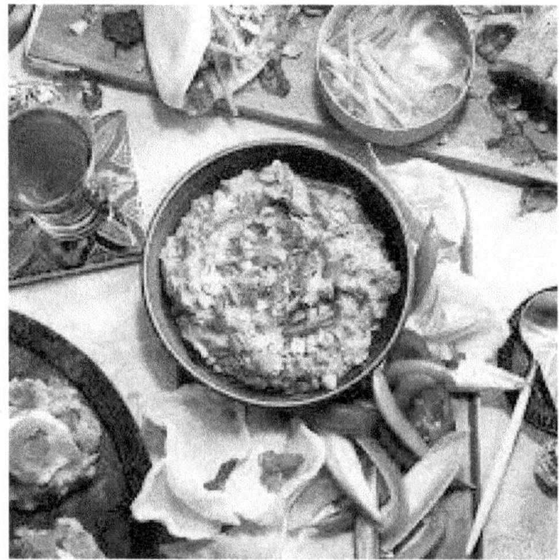

Preparation Time: 10 Minutes
Cooking Time: 30 Minutes
Serving 4
Ingredients:

- 1-pound Thai eggplant (or Japanese or Chinese eggplant)
- 2 tablespoons rice vinegar
- 2 teaspoons sugar
- 1 teaspoon low-sodium soy sauce
- 1 jalapeño pepper
- 2 garlic cloves
- ¼ cup chopped basil
- Cut vegetables or crackers, for serving

Direction:

1. Preheat the oven to 425°F.
2. Pierce the eggplant in several places with a skewer or knife. Place on a rimmed baking sheet and cook until soft,

about 30 minutes. Let cool, cut in half, and scoop out the flesh of the eggplant into a blender.

3. Add the rice vinegar, sugar, soy sauce, jalapeño, garlic, and basil to the blender. Process until smooth. Serve with cut vegetables or crackers.

Lower sodium tip: If you need to lower your sodium further, omit the soy sauce to lower the sodium to 3mg.
Nutrition: Per Serving Calories: 40; Total Fat: 0g; Saturated Fat: 0g; Cholesterol: 0mg; Carbohydrates: 10g; Fiber: 4g; Protein: 2g; Phosphorus: 34mg; Potassium: 284mg; Sodium: 47mg

44. Collard Salad Rolls with Peanut Dipping Sauce

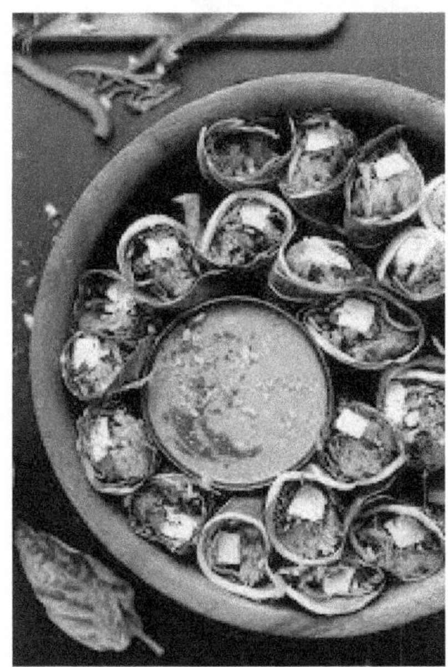

Preparation Time: 20 Minutes
Cooking Time:
Serving: 4
Ingredients:
For The Dipping Sauce

- ¼ cup peanut butter
- 2 tablespoons honey
- Juice of 1 lime
- ¼ teaspoon red chili flakes

For The Salad Rolls

- 4 ounces extra-firm tofu
- 1 bunch collard greens
- 1 cup thinly sliced purple cabbage
- 1 cup bean sprouts
- 2 carrots, cut into matchsticks
- ½ cup cilantro leaves and stems

Direction:
TO MAKE THE DIPPING SAUCE

1. In a blender, combine the peanut butter, honey, lime juice, and chili flakes, and process until smooth. Add 1 to 2 tablespoons of water as desired for consistency.

TO MAKE THE SALAD ROLLS

1. Using paper towels, press the excess moisture from the tofu. Cut into ½-inch-thick matchsticks.
2. Remove any tough stems from the collard greens and set aside.
3. Arrange all of the ingredients within reach. Cup one collard green leaf in your hand, and add a couple pieces of the tofu and a small amount each of the cabbage, bean sprouts, and carrots. Top with a couple cilantro sprigs, and roll into a cylinder. Place each roll, seam-side down, on a serving platter while you assemble the rest of the rolls. Serve with the dipping sauce.

Substitution tip: To lower the potassium, omit the cabbage and use only 1 carrot, which will drop the potassium to 208mg.

NutritionPer Serving Calories: 174; Total Fat: 9g; Saturated Fat: 2g; Cholesterol: 0mg; Carbohydrates: 20g; Fiber: 5g; Protein: 8g; Phosphorus: 56mg; Potassium: 284mg; Sodium: 42mg

45.   Simple Roasted Broccoli

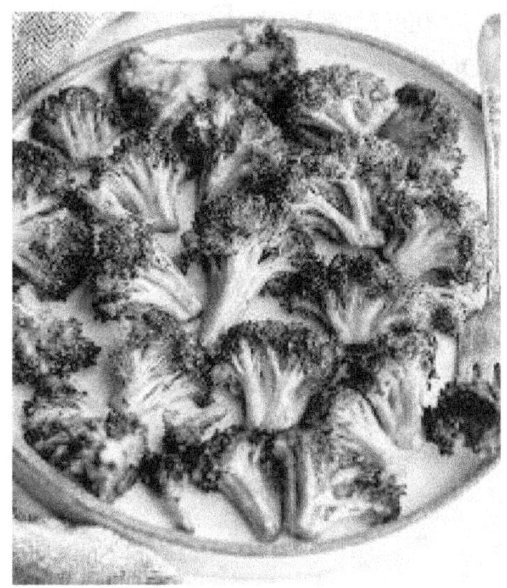

Preparation Time: 5 Minutes
Cooking Time: 20 Minutes
Serving: 6
Ingredients:

- 2 small heads broccoli, cut into florets
- 1 tablespoon extra-virgin olive oil
- 3 garlic cloves, minced

Direction:

1. Preheat the oven to 425°F.
2. In a medium bowl, toss the broccoli with the olive oil and garlic. Arrange in a single layer on a baking sheet

3. 3Roast for 10 minutes, then flip the broccoli and roast an additional 10 minutes. Serve.

Cooking tip: Roasted broccoli makes for great leftovers—throw them in a quick salad for added flavor and bulk. To save leftovers, refrigerate in an airtight container for three to five days.
Nutrition Per Serving Calories: 38; Total Fat: 2g; Saturated Fat: 0g; Cholesterol: 0mg; Carbohydrates: 4g; Fiber: 1g; Protein: 1g; Phosphorus: 32mg; Potassium: 150mg; Sodium: 15mg

46.   Roasted Mint Carrots

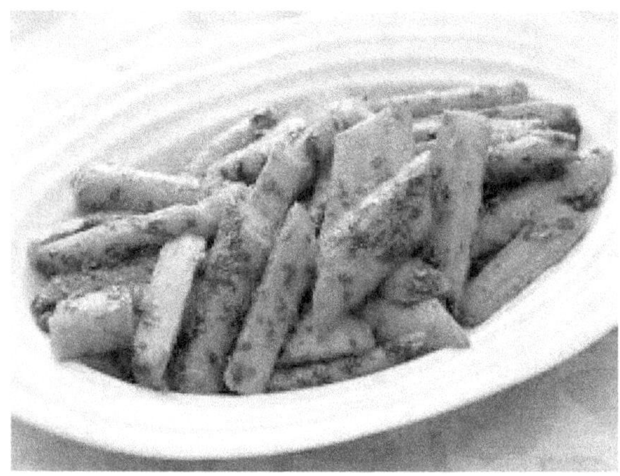

Preparation Time: 5 Minutes
Cooking Time: 20 Minutes
Serving: 6
Ingredients:

- 1-pound carrots, trimmed
- 1 tablespoon extra-virgin olive oil
- Freshly ground black pepper
- ¼ cup thinly sliced mint

Direction:

1. Preheat the oven to 425°F.

2. Arrange the carrots in a single layer on a rimmed baking sheet. Drizzle with the olive oil, and shake the carrots on the sheet to coat. Season with pepper.
3. Roast for 20 minutes, or until tender and browned, stirring twice while cooking. Sprinkle with the mint and serve.

Substitution tip: To lower the potassium in this dish, use 8 ounces of carrots and 8 ounces of turnips cut into cubes. This will cut the potassium to 193mg.

Nutrition Per Serving Calories: 51; Total Fat: 2g; Saturated Fat: 0g; Cholesterol: 0mg; Carbohydrates: 7g; Fiber: 2g; Protein: 1g; Phosphorus: 26mg; Potassium: 242mg; Sodium: 52mg

47.   Roasted Root Vegetables

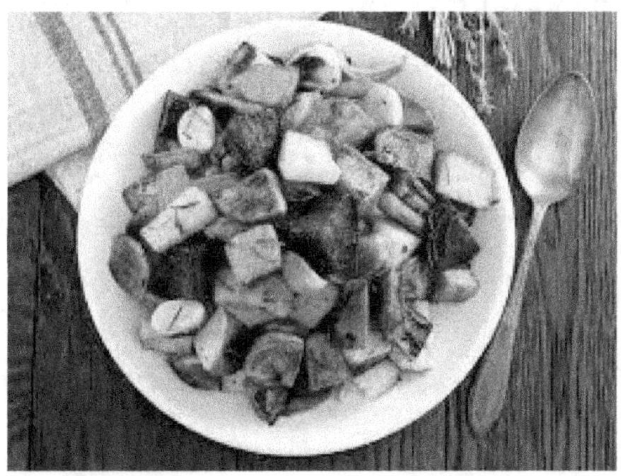

Preparation Time: 10 Minutes
Cooking Time: 25 Minutes
Serving: 6
Ingredients:

- 1 cup chopped turnips
- 1 cup chopped rutabaga
- 1 cup chopped parsnips
- 1 tablespoon extra-virgin olive oil
- 1 teaspoon fresh chopped rosemary

- Freshly ground black pepper

Direction:

1. Preheat the oven to 400°F.
2. In a large bowl, toss the turnips, rutabaga, and parsnips with the olive oil and rosemary. Arrange in a single layer on a baking sheet, and season with pepper.
3. Bake until the vegetables are tender and browned, 20 to 25 minutes, stirring once.

Substitution tip: Experiment with other fresh herbs in this dish to suit your own tastes. Thyme, tarragon, oregano, and minced garlic all add unique flavors to these root vegetables.

Nutrition Per Serving Calories: 52; Total Fat: 2g; Saturated Fat: 0g; Cholesterol: 0mg; Carbohydrates: 7g; Fiber: 2g; Protein: 1g; Phosphorus: 35mg; Potassium: 205mg; Sodium: 22mg

48. Vegetable Couscous

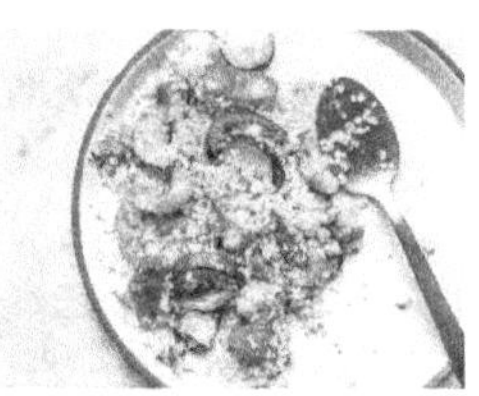

Preparation Time: 10 Minutes
Cooking Time: 15 Minutes
Serving: 6
Ingredients:

- 1 tablespoon extra-virgin olive oil
- ½ sweet onion, diced
- 1 carrot, diced
- 1 celery stalk, diced
- ½ cup diced red or yellow bell pepper

- 1 small zucchini, diced
- 1 cup couscous
- 1½ cups Simple Chicken Broth or low-sodium store-bought chicken stock
- ½ teaspoon garlic powder
- Freshly ground black pepper

Direction:

1. In a large skillet, heat the olive oil over medium heat. Add the onion, carrot, celery, and bell pepper, and cook, stirring occasionally, until the vegetables are just becoming tender, about 5 to 7 minutes.
2. Add the zucchini, couscous, broth, and garlic powder. Stir to blend, and bring to a boil. Cover and remove from the heat. Let stand for 5 to 8 minutes. Fluff with a fork, season with pepper, and serve.

Substitution tip: Swap out vegetables to make this couscous your own creation. Yellow summer squash or pattypan squash can be substituted for the zucchini. Other vegetables, like asparagus, broccoli, or cauliflower, can be added instead of carrots and bell peppers.

Nutrition Per Serving Calories: 154; Total Fat: 3g; Saturated Fat: 1g; Cholesterol: 0mg; Carbohydrates: 27g; Fiber: 2g; Protein: 5g; Phosphorus: 83mg; Potassium: 197mg; Sodium: 36mg

49. Garlic Cauliflower Rice

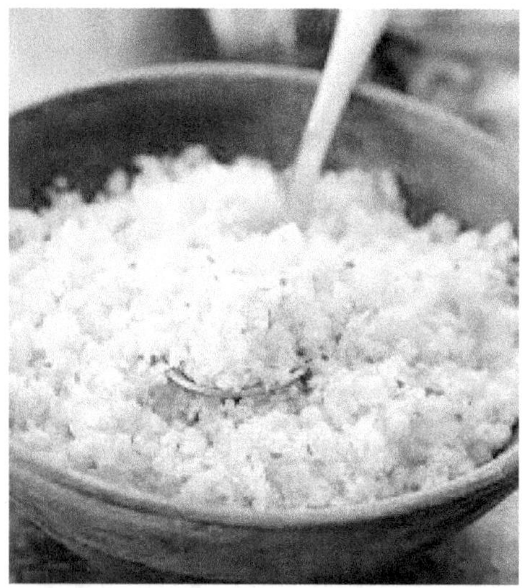

Preparation Time: 5 Minutes
Cooking Time: 10 Minutes
Serving: 8

Ingredients:

- 1 medium head cauliflower
- 1 tablespoon extra-virgin olive oil
- 4 garlic cloves, minced
- Freshly ground black pepper

Direction:

1. Using a sharp knife, remove the core of the cauliflower, and separate the cauliflower into florets.
2. In a food processor, pulse the florets until they are the size of rice, being careful not to over process them to the point of becoming mushy.
3. In a large skillet over medium heat, heat the olive oil. Add the garlic, and stir until just fragrant.
4. Add the cauliflower, stirring to coat. Add 1 tablespoon of water to the pan, cover, and reduce the heat to low. Steam

for 7 to 10 minutes, until the cauliflower is tender. Season with pepper and serve.

Cooking tip: Cauliflower rice tastes great both when fresh and after resting in the refrigerator for a day or two. Make a batch and use it throughout the week as a side dish, heating it in the microwave before serving. In an airtight container, it will keep refrigerated for three to five days.

Nutrition Per Serving Calories: 37; Total Fat: 2g; Saturated Fat: 0g; Cholesterol: 0mg; Carbohydrates: 4g; Fiber: 2g; Protein: 2g; Phosphorus: 35mg; Potassium: 226mg; Sodium: 22mg

50. Veggie Snack

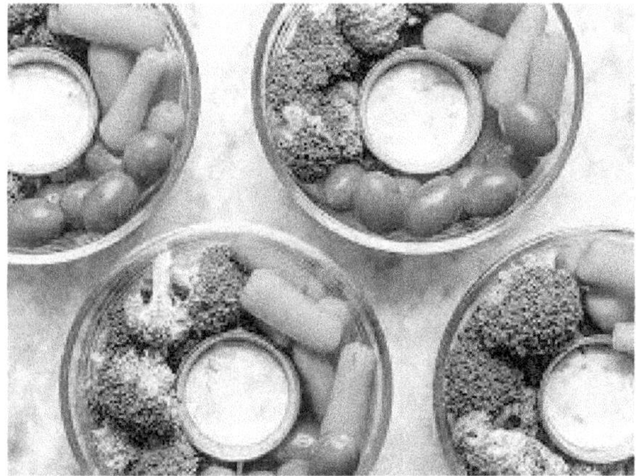

Preparation Time: 5 minutes
Cooking Time: 10 minutes
Servings: 1
Ingredients:

- 1 large yellow pepper
- 5 carrots
- 5 stalks celery

Directions:

1. Clean the carrots and rinse under running water.
2. Rinse celery and yellow pepper. Remove seeds of pepper and chop the veggies into small sticks.
3. Put in a bowl and serve.

Nutrition: Calories: 189 Fat: 0.5 g Carbs: 44.3 g Protein: 5 g Sodium: 282 mg Potassium: 0mg Phosphorus: 0mg

51.   Roasted Asparagus

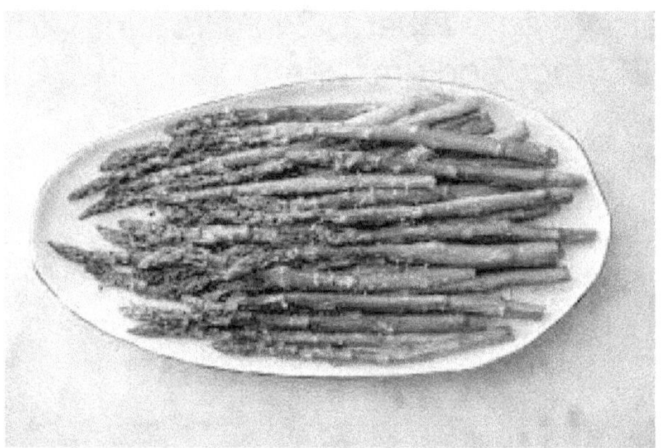

Preparation Time: 5 minutes
Cooking Time: 10 minutes
Servings: 4
Ingredients:

- 1 tbsp. extra virgin olive oil
- 1-pound fresh asparagus
- 1 medium lemon, zested
- 1/2 tsp. freshly grated nutmeg
- 1/2 tsp. kosher salt
- ½ tsp. black pepper

Directions:

1. Preheat your oven to 500 degrees F.

2. Put asparagus on an aluminum foil and add extra virgin olive oil.
3. Prepare asparagus in a single layer and fold the edges of the foil.
4. Cook in the oven for 5 minutes. Continue roasting until browned.
5. Add the roasted asparagus with nutmeg, salt, zest, and pepper before serving.

Nutrition: Calories: 55 Fat: 3.8 g Carbs: 4.7 g Protein: 2.5 g Sodium: 98mg Potassium: 172mg Phosphorus: 35mg

52. Cinnamon Apple Fries

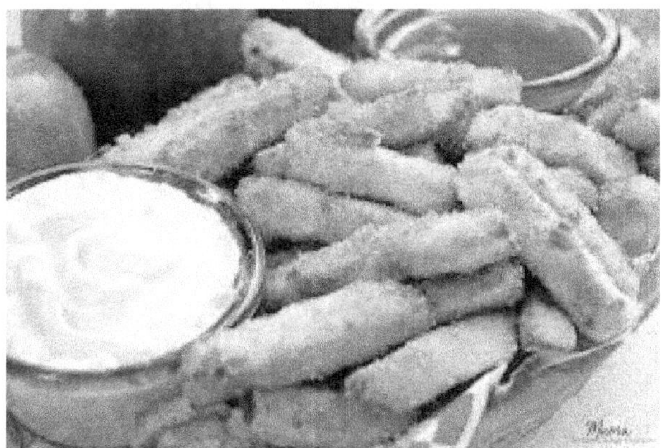

Preparation Time: 5 minutes
Cooking Time: 15 minutes
Servings: 1
Ingredients:

- 1 apple, sliced thinly
- Dash of cinnamon
- Stevia

Directions:

1. Coat apple slices with cinnamon and stevia.
2. Bake for 15 minutes or until tender and crispy at 325 degrees F.

Nutrition: Calories: 146 Fat: 0.7 g Carbs: 36.4 g Protein: 1.6 g Sodium: 10 mg Potassium: 100mg Phosphorus: 0mg

53. Vinegar & Salt Kale

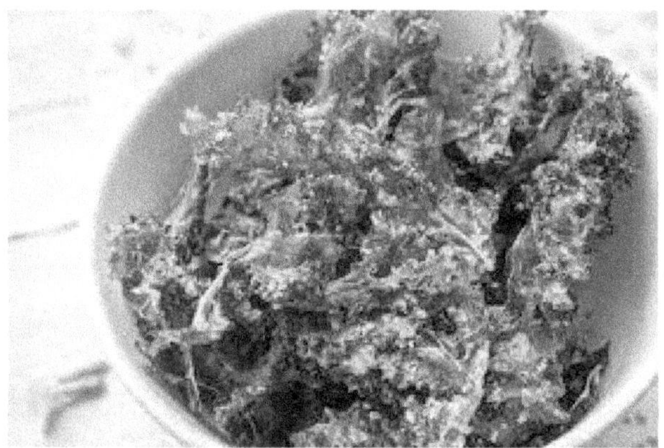

Preparation Time: 10 minutes
Cooking Time: 12 minutes
Servings: 2
Ingredients:

- 1 head kale, chopped
- 1 teaspoon extra virgin olive oil
- 1 tablespoon apple cider vinegar
- ½ teaspoon of sea salt

Directions:

1. Prepare kale in a bowl and put vinegar and extra virgin olive oil.
2. Sprinkle with salt and massage the ingredients with hands.

3. Spread the kale out onto two paper-lined baking sheets and bake at 375°F for about 12 minutes or until crispy.
4. Let cool for about 10 minutes before serving.

Nutrition: Calories: 152 Fat: 8.2 g Carbs: 15.2 g Protein: 4 g Sodium: 170mg Potassium: 304mg Phosphorus: 37mg

<u>Are you enjoying this book? If so, I'd be genuinely happy if you could leave a short review on Amazon, it actually helps!</u>

Thank you.

54. <u>Lemon Pops</u>

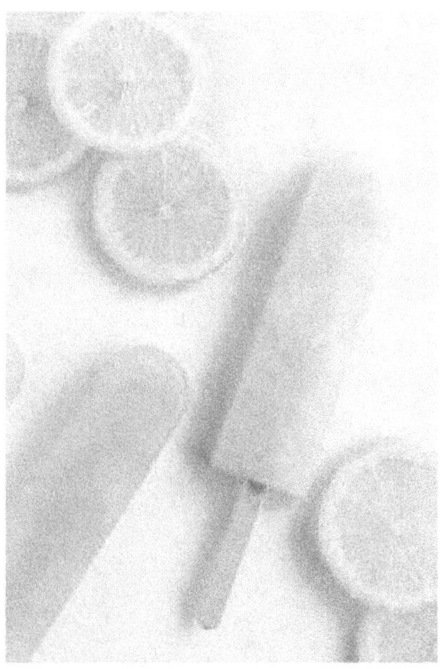

Preparation Time: 5 minutes
Cooking Time: 5 minutes
Servings: 1
Ingredients:

- 4 tablespoons fresh lemon juice
- Powdered stevia

Directions:

1. Mix mango or lemon juice and stevia and pour into molds.
2. Freeze until firm.

Nutrition: Calories: 46 Fat: 0.2g Carbs: 16g Protein: 0.9g Sodium: 3.7mg Potassium: 104mg Phosphorus: 11mg

55. Apple & Strawberry Snack

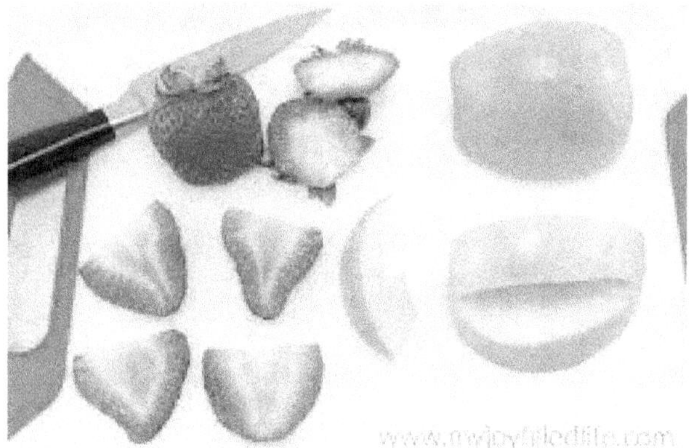

Preparation Time: 5 minutes
Cooking Time: 2 minutes
Servings: 1
Ingredients:

- ½ apple, cored and sliced
- 2-3 strawberries
- dash of ground cinnamon
- 2-3 drops stevia 2-3 drops

Directions:

1. In a bowl, mix strawberries and apples and sprinkle with
   stevia and cinnamon.
2. Microwave for about 1-2 minutes. Serve warm.

Nutrition: Calories: 145 Fat: 0.8 g Carbs: 34.2 g Protein: 1.6 g
Sodium: 20 mg Potassium: 0mg Phosphorus: 0mg

56. Candied Macadamia Nuts

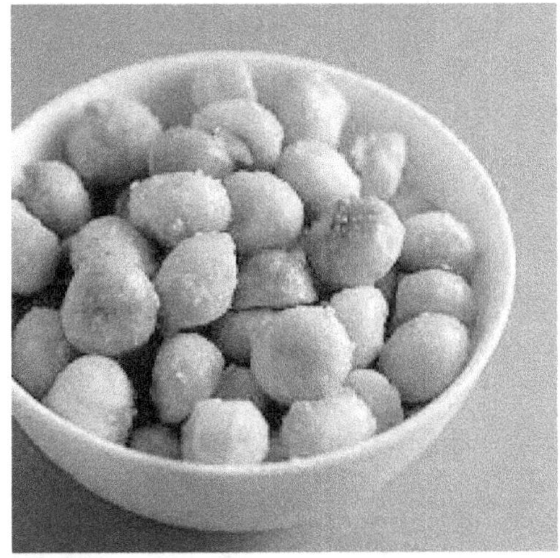

Preparation Time: 5 minutes
Cooking Time: 15 minutes
Servings: 2
Ingredients:

- 2 cups macadamia nuts
- 1 tablespoon extra-virgin olive oil
- 2 tablespoons honey

Directions:

1. Toss ingredients in bowl and spread into a baking dish.
2. Bake for 15 minutes at 350°F.
3. Let cool before serving.

Nutrition: Calories: 200 Fat: 18 g Carbs: 10g Protein: 1g Sodium: 5 mg Potassium: 55mg Phosphorus: 10mg

57.   Healthy Spiced Nuts

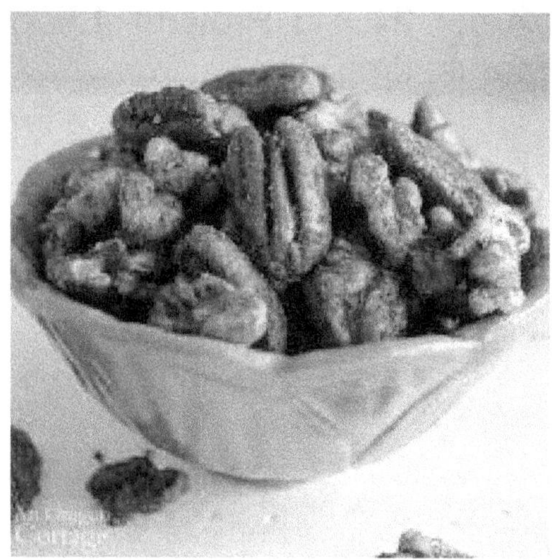

Preparation Time: 10 minutes
Cooking Time: 10 minutes
Servings: 4
Ingredients:

- 1 tbsp. extra virgin olive oil
- ¼ cup walnuts
- ¼ cup pecans
- ¼ cup almonds
- ½ tsp. sea salt
- ½ tsp. cumin
- ½ tsp. pepper
- 1 tsp. chili powder

Directions:

1. Put the skillet on medium heat and toast the nuts until lightly browned.

2. Prepare the spice mixture and add black pepper, cumin, chili, and salt.
3. Put extra virgin olive oil and sprinkle with spice mixture to the toasted nuts before serving.

Nutrition: Calories: 88 Fat: 8g Carbs: 4g Protein: 2.5g Sodium: 51mgPotassium: 88mg
Phosphorus: 6.3mg

58.   Low-Fat Mango Salsa

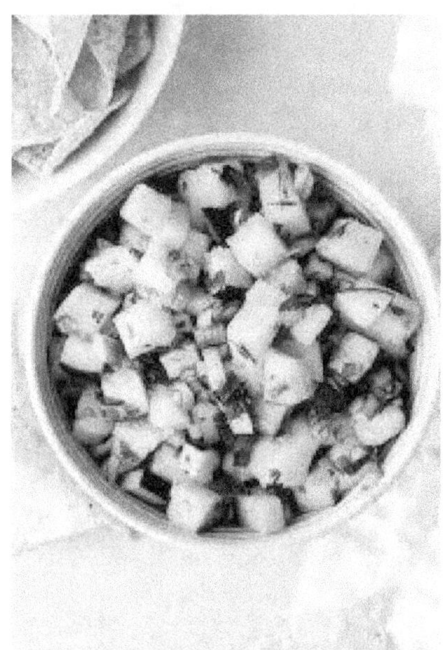

Preparation Time: 10 minutes
Cooking Time: 10 minutes
Servings: 4
Ingredients:

- 1 cup cucumber, chopped
- 2 cups mango, diced
- ½ cup cilantro, minced
- 2 tablespoons fresh lime juice

- 1 tablespoon scallions, minced
- ¼ teaspoon chipotle powder
- ¼ teaspoon sea salt

Directions

1. Mix the ingredients in a bowl and serve or refrigerate.

Nutrition: Calories: 155 Fat: 0.6 g Carbs: 38.2 g Protein: 1.4 g Sodium: 3.2 mg Potassium: 221mg Phosphorus: 27mg

59.   Easy No-Bake Coconut Cookies

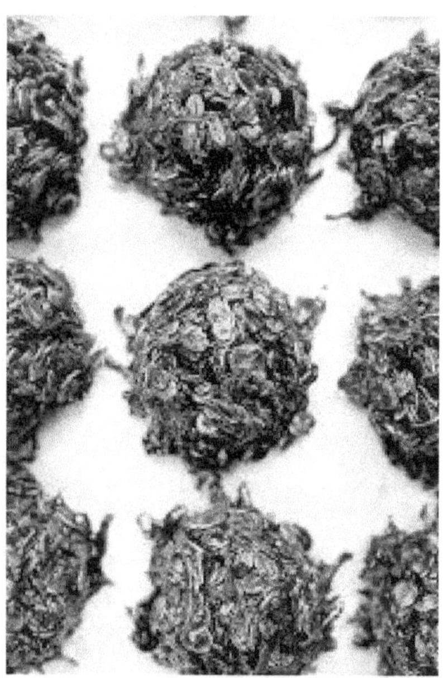

Preparation Time: 5 minutes
Cooking Time: 10 minutes
Servings: 20
Ingredients:

- 3 cups finely shredded coconut flakes
- 1 cup melted coconut oil
- 1 teaspoon liquid stevia

Directions:

1. Prepare all ingredients in a large bowl; stir until well blended.
2. Form the mixture into small balls and arrange them on a paper-lined baking tray.
3. Press each cookie down with a fork and refrigerate until firm. Enjoy!

Nutrition: Calories: 99 Fat: 10 g Carbs: 2 g Protein: 3 Sodium: 7 m
Potassium: 105mg
Phosphorus: 11mg

60. Vegetable Bisque

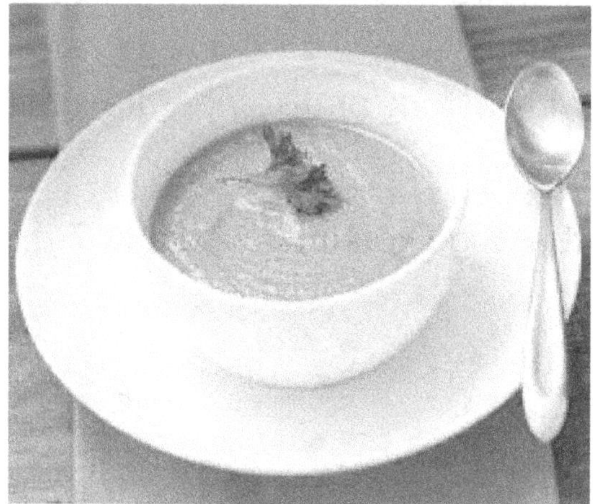

Preparation Time: 15 minutes
Cooking Time: 30 minutes
Serving: 4

Ingredients:

- 4 cups low-sodium vegetable broth
- 3 large carrots, sliced
- 1 yellow bell pepper, sliced
- 1 cup sliced button mushrooms
- 1/8 teaspoon salt
- 1/8 teaspoon freshly ground black pepper
- 1 (8-ounce) package cream cheese, cubed

Direction:

1. 1.In a heavy saucepan, combine the broth, carrots, bell pepper, mushrooms, salt, and pepper over medium heat. Bring to a boil, then reduce the heat to low.

2. 2.Simmer for 20 to 25 minutes, or until the vegetables are very tender.
3. 3.Using a slotted spoon, remove the vegetables from the broth and transfer them to a food processor. Add the cream cheese and process until smooth.
4. 4.Return the pureed mixture to the broth in the saucepan and stir. Reheat for 3 to 5 minutes, until steaming. Do not boil. Serve.
5. Appliance Tip: You can cook this soup in the slow cooker. Combine the mushrooms, carrots, broth, salt, and pepper in a 3-quart slow cooker. Cover and cook on low for 6 to 8 hours or until the vegetables are tender. Puree the vegetables in a food processor with the cream cheese and cream as directed above, then return to the slow cooker. Heat on high for 30 minutes, then serve.

Nutrition Per Serving Calories: 247; Total fat: 20g; Saturated fat: 12g; Sodium: 429mg; Phosphorus: 109mg; Potassium: 386mg; Carbohydrates: 14g; Fiber: 2g; Protein: 5g; Sugar: 7g

61.   French Onion Soup

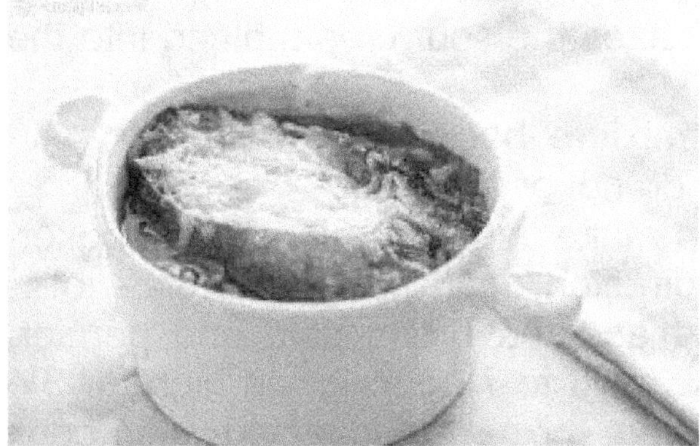

Preparation Time: 25 minutes
Cooking Time: 70 minutes
Serving: 4

Ingredients:

- 2 tablespoons butter
- 1 tablespoon extra-virgin olive oil
- 3 large yellow onions, chopped
- 5 cups low-sodium vegetable broth
- 1/8 teaspoon salt
- 1/8 teaspoon freshly ground black pepper
- 1 cup sour cream
- 2 tablespoons cornstarch

Direction:

1. In a large saucepan, melt the butter with the olive oil over medium heat. Add the onions, reduce the heat to medium low, and cook for about 30 minutes, stirring occasionally, until the onions are golden brown.
2. .Add the broth, salt, and pepper and bring to a simmer. Simmer for 20 to 30 minutes.
3. .In a medium bowl, whisk the sour cream and cornstarch.
4. 4.Add 1 cup of the hot broth from the soup to the sour cream mixture and whisk together until smooth. This is called tempering and makes the sour cream blend into the soup without curdling.
5. .Add the sour cream mixture back to the soup and stir. Reheat until steaming; do not boil. Serve.
6. Appliance Tip: You can make this recipe in a slow cooker. Brown the onions as directed, then transfer to a 3- to 4-quart slow cooker and add the broth, salt, and pepper. Cover and cook on low for 6 to 7 hours or on high for 3½ hours. Add the sour cream mixture as directed, then cook on high for 20 to 30 minutes or until hot.

Nutrition Per Serving Calories: 269; Total fat: 21g; Saturated fat: 10g; Sodium: 314mg; Phosphorus: 87mg; Potassium: 292mg; Carbohydrates: 20g; Fiber: 2g; Protein: 3g; Sugar: 8g

62.   Tomato-Free Slow Cooker White Chili

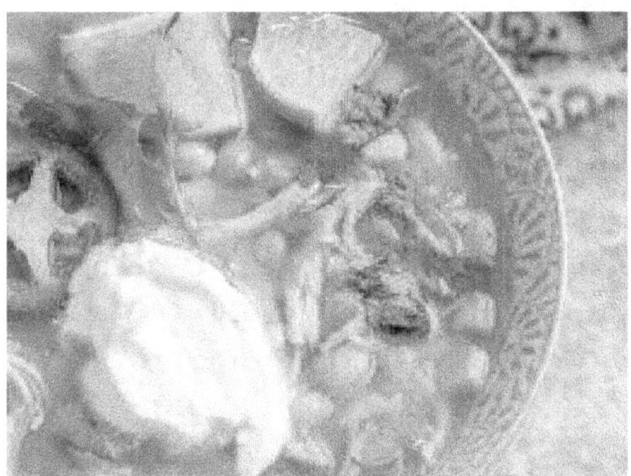

Preparation Time: 20 minutes
Cooking Time: 8 hours
Serving: 6
Ingredients:

- 1 cup dried kidney beans, sorted and rinsed
- 6 cups low-sodium vegetable broth
- 1 yellow onion, chopped
- 4 garlic cloves, minced
- 2 tablespoons chili powder
- 1/8 teaspoon salt
- 1/8 teaspoon freshly ground black pepper
- 2 tablespoons extra-virgin olive oil

Direction:

1. In a large saucepan, cover the beans with water and bring to a boil. Boil for 10 minutes. Drain the beans, discarding the water.

2. .In a 4-quart slow cooker, combine the beans, broth, onion, garlic, chili powder, salt, and pepper.
3. .Cover and cook on low for 6 to 8 hours or on high for 3 to 4 hours, or until the beans and rice are tender.
4. .Transfer ½ cup of the beans from the slow cooker to a food processor or blender. Add the olive oil and puree. Return to the slow cooker. Heat on high for 20 minutes, then serve.
5. Appliance Tip: You can make this recipe on the stovetop. Boil the beans as directed, drain, then cover with fresh water again and bring to a simmer. Remove the pan from the heat and let the beans soak for 1 hour. Drain the beans again, then add all the remaining ingredients. Partially cover and simmer for 1½ hours or until the beans are tender.

Nutrition Per Serving Calories: 171; Total fat: 5g; Saturated fat: 1g; Sodium: 271mg; Phosphorus: 148mg; Potassium: 561mg; Carbohydrates: 24g; Fiber: 9g; Protein: 8g; Sugar: 3g

63. Minestrone

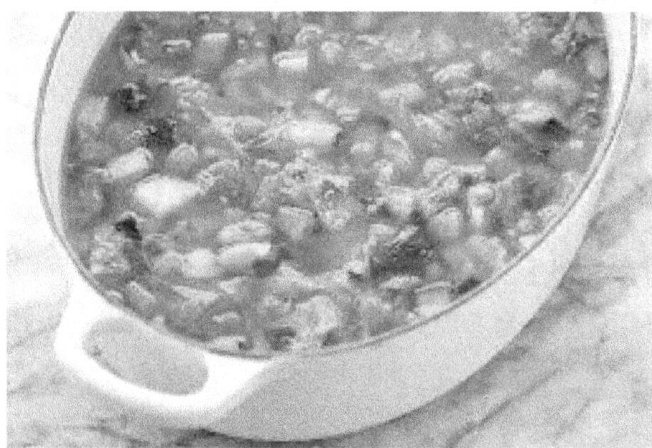

Preparation Time: 20 minutes
Cooking Time: 35 minutes
Serving: 4

Ingredients:

- 2 tablespoons extra-virgin olive oil
- 1 yellow onion, chopped
- 2 large carrots, peeled and chopped
- 4 cups low-sodium vegetable broth
- 2 cups green beans, cut into 2-inch pieces
- 1/8 teaspoon salt
- 1/8 teaspoon freshly ground black pepper
- ½ cup whole-wheat orzo pasta

Direction:

1. 1.In a large saucepan, heat the olive oil over medium heat.
2. 2.Add the onion and cook for 3 to 4 minutes, stirring, until the onion starts to soften.
3. 3.Add the carrots, cook, and stir for another 3 minutes.
4. 4.Add the broth, green beans, salt, and pepper and bring to a simmer.
5. 5.Reduce the heat to low and simmer for 15 to 20 minutes or until the vegetables are almost tender.
6. 6.Add the pasta and bring back to a simmer. Simmer for 8 to 10 minutes or until the pasta is tender. Serve.
7. Increase Protein Tip: To make this a high-protein recipe, use low-sodium chicken broth instead of vegetable broth. The protein content will increase to 10 grams per serving.
8. Ingredient Tip: You can serve this recipe topped with Easy Pesto or top with some grated Parmesan cheese for the perfect finishing touch.

Nutrition Per Serving Calories: 190; Total fat: 8g; Saturated fat: 1g; Sodium: 243mg; Phosphorus: 113g; Potassium: 354mg; Carbohydrates: 27g; Fiber: 5g; Protein: 5g; Sugar: 5g

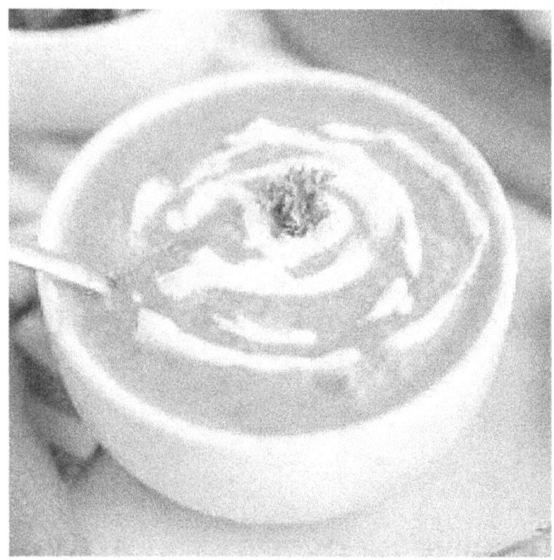

Preparation Time: 20 minutes
Cooking Time: 50 minutes
Serving: 4

Ingredients:

- 6 large carrots, peeled and sliced
- 1 red onion, chopped
- 2 tablespoons extra-virgin olive oil
- 1 tablespoon minced peeled fresh ginger
- 1/8 teaspoon salt
- 1/8 teaspoon freshly ground black pepper
- 3½ cups water
- ½ cup pineapple-orange juice
- ½ cup sour cream

Direction:

1. 1.Preheat the oven to 400°F.
2. 2.On a large rimmed baking sheet, place the carrots and onion and drizzle with the olive oil. Sprinkle with the ginger,

salt, and pepper. Toss to coat.

3. 3.Roast the vegetables for 30 to 35 minutes, stirring twice while they cook, until they are tender and lightly browned around the edges.
4. 4.Transfer the vegetables to a large saucepan. Add the water and bring to a simmer. Simmer for 10 minutes or until the vegetables are soft.
5. 5.In a food processor, puree the mixture in three separate batches because hot soup expands when blended. Return to the saucepan.
6. 6.In a medium bowl, combine the pineapple-orange juice and sour cream and whisk together. Add 1 cup of the hot soup and whisk again. Stir into the soup and heat through; serve.
7. Ingredient Tip: To make this recipe vegan, omit the sour cream and add richness by topping the soup with a tablespoon of coconut cream. Coconut cream is available canned in most grocery stores.

Nutrition Per Serving Calories: 173; Total fat: 13g; Saturated fat: 4g; Sodium: 315mg; Phosphorus: 68mg; Potassium: 429mg; Carbohydrates: 15g; Fiber: 4g; Protein: 2g; Sugar: 7g

65.   Roasted Onion Clam Chowder

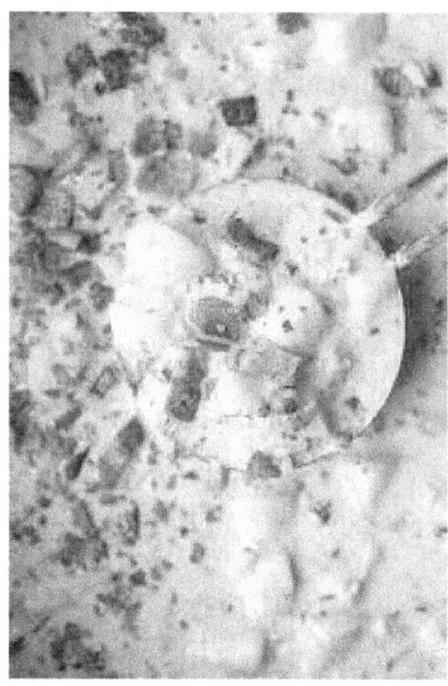

Preparation Time: 20 minutes
Cooking Time: 1 hour
Serving: 6
Ingredients:

- 2 russet potatoes, peeled and cubed
- 2 yellow onions, chopped
- 8 whole unpeeled garlic cloves
- 2 tablespoons extra-virgin olive oil
- 4 cups low-sodium chicken stock
- 1/8 teaspoon salt
- 1/8 teaspoon freshly ground black pepper
- 1 (10-ounce) can clams

Direction:

1. 1.Place the potatoes in a large saucepan, cover with water, and bring to a boil on high heat. Boil for 10 minutes, then drain the potatoes and discard the water.
2. 2.Preheat the oven to 400°F.

3. 3.On a rimmed baking sheet, combine the onions, garlic, and olive oil. Roast for 30 to 35 minutes, stirring once during the cooking time, until they are tender and light golden brown around the edges. Squeeze the garlic to remove the skins. Discard the skins and set the garlic and onions aside.
4. 4.In the same saucepan, combine the potatoes, chicken stock, salt, and pepper and bring to a boil over medium heat. Reduce the heat to low and simmer for 20 to 25 minutes or until the potatoes are tender.
5. 5.Using a potato masher, mash half of the potatoes, leaving some whole for a chunky texture.
6. 6.Add the onions and garlic to the saucepan along with the clams and their juices. Simmer for 5 to 10 minutes or until hot. Serve.
7. Diabetes Tip: To make this a diabetes-friendly recipe, omit the potatoes, skip step 1, and use 2 parsnips instead. The carbohydrate content will decrease to 18g per serving.

Nutrition Per Serving Calories: 216; Total fat: 6g; Saturated fat: 1g; Sodium: 141mg; Phosphorus: 205mg; Potassium: 565mg; Carbohydrates: 29g; Fiber: 3g; Protein: 13g; Sugar: 3g

66. Chicken Parmesan Soup

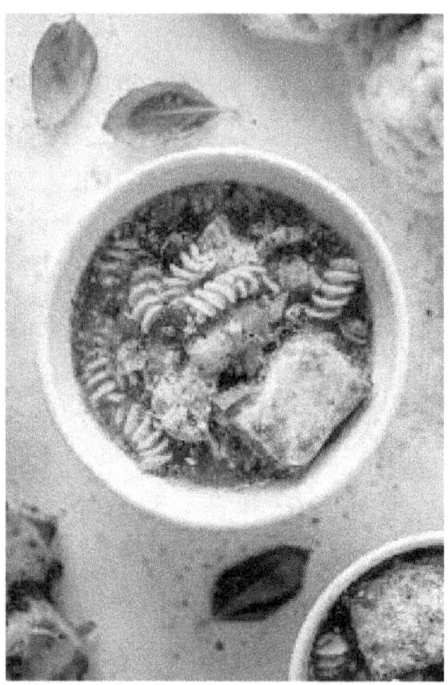

Preparation Time: 20 minutes
Cooking Time: 7 hours
Serving: 4
Ingredients:

- 1 leek, chopped
- 2 tablespoons extra-virgin olive oil
- 2 (6-ounce) bone-in, skin-on chicken breasts
- 2 cups frozen corn
- 4 cups water, divided
- 2 tablespoons tomato paste
- 1/8 teaspoon salt
- 1/8 teaspoon freshly ground black pepper
- 3 tablespoons grated Parmesan cheese

Direction:

1. 1.Place the leek in a 3- to 4-quart slow cooker.
2. 2.In a large saucepan, heat the olive oil over medium heat. Add the chicken breasts, skin-side down, and cook for 8 to

10 minutes, until well-browned.

3. 3.Place the chicken in the slow cooker and top with the corn.
4. 4.In the same saucepan used to brown the chicken, combine 1 cup of water and the tomato paste and bring to a simmer, scraping up the brown bits. Pour into the slow cooker along with the remaining 3 cups of water, the salt, and pepper.
5. 5.Cover and cook on low for 6 to 7 hours.
6. 6.Remove the chicken from the soup and let cool for 15 minutes. Remove the skin and bones and discard. Shred the chicken, then return it to the soup.
7. 7.Cook on high for 10 minutes, then serve topped with cheese.
8. Ingredient Tip: Feel free to add more fresh or dried herbs or spices to this recipe. Basil, oregano, and parsley are all excellent possibilities.

Nutrition Per Serving Calories: 323; Total fat: 15g; Saturated fat: 4g; Sodium: 226mg; Phosphorus: 233mg; Potassium: 441mg; Carbohydrates: 21g; Fiber: 3g; Protein: 28g; Sugar: 5g

67. Slow Cooker Potato Leek Soup

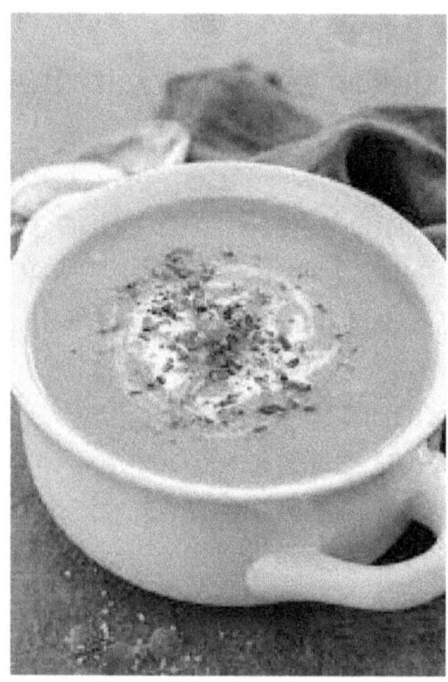

Preparation Time: 15 minutes
Cooking Time: 8 hours
Serving: 4
Ingredients:

- 2 large russet potatoes, peeled and chopped
- 5 cups low-sodium chicken broth
- 2 leeks, rinsed and chopped
- 1/8 teaspoon salt
- 1/8 teaspoon freshly ground black pepper
- 1 cup heavy cream
- 2 tablespoons minced chives

Direction:

1. 1.Place the potatoes in a large saucepan, cover with water, and bring to a boil on high heat. Boil for 10 minutes, then drain the potatoes and discard the water.
2. 2.In the slow cooker, combine the potatoes, broth, leeks, salt, and pepper. Cover and cook on low for 6 to 8 hours.

3. 3.Add the cream to the slow cooker. Using an immersion blender or potato masher, blend or mash the vegetables to make a smooth soup. You can also puree the vegetables in a food processor; do them half at a time, then return to the slow cooker.
4. 4.Heat the soup for 20 minutes on high, then serve, garnished with the chives.
5. Ingredient Tip: Leeks can be very sandy, so after you cut off the root end and about 3 inches of the green part, cut the leeks in half. Rinse them under cool, running water, making sure to separate the leaves to get out all the sand. Then chop and continue with the recipe.
6. Reduce Protein Tip: To make this a medium-protein recipe, replace the chicken broth with low-sodium vegetable broth. The protein content will decrease to 7g per serving.

Nutrition Per Serving Calories: 395; Total fat: 24g; Saturated fat: 14g; Sodium: 201mg; Phosphorus: 243mg; Potassium: 599mg; Carbohydrates: 45g; Fiber: 3g; Protein: 12g; Sugar: 5g

68. Thai-Style Beet Soup

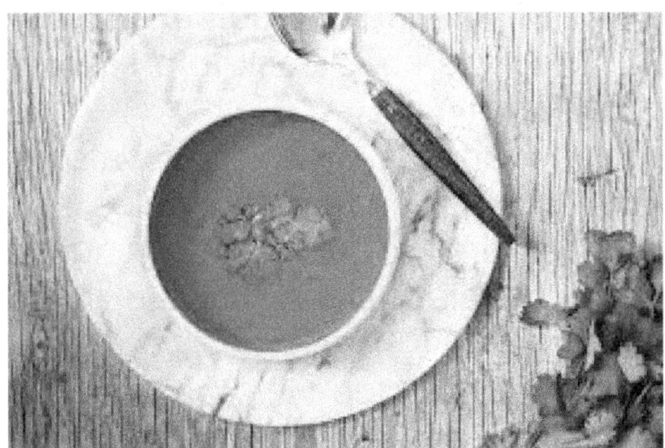

Preparation Time: 15 minutes
Cooking Time: 35 minutes
Serving: 4

Ingredients:

- 2 tablespoons extra-virgin olive oil
- 3 medium beets, scrubbed, peeled, and chopped
- 5 cups water
- 2 tablespoons yellow curry paste
- 1/8 teaspoon salt
- 1/8 teaspoon freshly ground black pepper
- 8 ounces thin rice noodles
- 1 lime, zested and juiced
- 3 tablespoons chopped fresh cilantro

Direction:

1. 1.In a large saucepan, heat the olive oil over medium heat.
2. 2.Add the beets and cook for 3 to 4 minutes while stirring. Add the water and yellow curry paste. Bring to a boil over medium heat. Then cover the pan, reduce the heat to low, and simmer for about 25 minutes, until the beets are tender.
3. 3.In a food processor, puree the soup in two or three batches or use an immersion blender or potato masher directly in the saucepan. Bring the soup back to a simmer over low heat, stirring occasionally.
4. 4.To prepare the rice noodles, bring a large pot of water to a boil over high heat. Using tongs, add the noodles and submerge. When the noodles are tender, 1 to 2 minutes, drain. If you are using flat noodles, it may take 8 to 10 minutes for the noodles to soften.
5. 5.Divide the soup among bowls and top with the noodles. Drizzle with the lime juice and zest, and sprinkle with the cilantro before serving.

Nutrition Per Serving Calories: 302; Total fat: 7g; Saturated fat: 1g; Sodium: 364mg; Phosphorus: 119mg; Potassium: 268mg; Carbohydrates: 54g; Fiber: 3g; Protein: 5g; Sugar: 5g

69.   Turkey and Corn Chowder

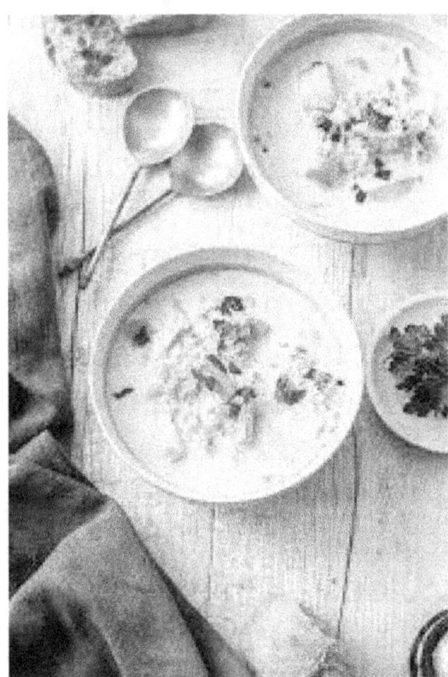

Preparation Time: 20 minutes
Cooking Time: 35 minutes
Serving: 6
Ingredients:

- 2 russet potatoes, peeled and chopped
- 2 tablespoons extra-virgin olive oil
- 1 onion, chopped
- 4 cups water
- 1½ cups frozen yellow corn
- 1/8 teaspoon salt
- 1/8 teaspoon freshly ground black pepper
- 2 cups shredded cooked turkey or chicken
- 1 cup heavy cream

Direction:

1. 1.Place the potatoes in a large saucepan, cover with water, and bring to a boil on high heat. Boil for 10 minutes, then drain the potatoes and discard the water.
2. 2.In a large saucepan, heat the olive oil over medium heat. Add the onion and cook for 3 to 4 minutes, stirring until tender.
3. 3.Add the water, corn, potatoes, salt, and pepper and bring to a simmer.
4. 4.Reduce the heat to low and simmer for 20 to 25 minutes or until the potatoes are tender. Remove half the vegetables from the soup and puree. Return to the soup.
5. 5.Add the turkey and cream to the soup. Heat over medium heat until steaming; do not boil. Serve.
6. Appliance Tip: You can make this recipe in the slow cooker. Boil the potatoes as directed, then omit the oil. Combine the onion, corn, water, potatoes, salt, and pepper in a 3- or 4- quart slow cooker. Cover and cook on low for 6 hours or on high for 3 hours. Then mash about half the veggies in the crockpot, add the cream and turkey, and heat on high for 10 minutes.

Nutrition Per Serving Calories: 307; Total fat: 20g; Saturated fat: 10g; Sodium: 110mg; Phosphorus: 181mg; Potassium: 407mg; Carbohydrates: 16g; Fiber: 2g; Protein: 17g; Sugar: 3g

70.   Hearty Veggie Stew

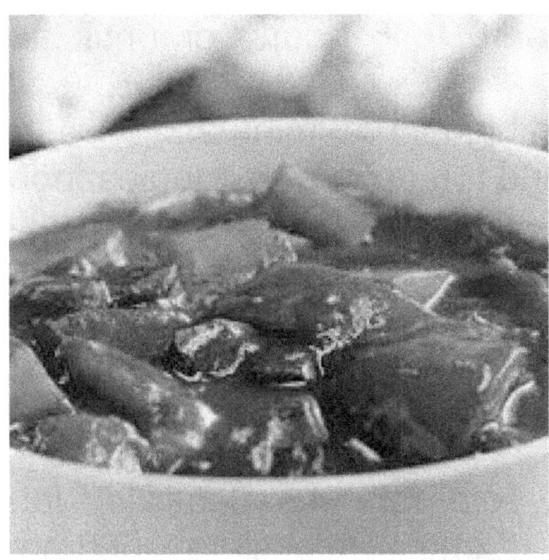

Preparation Time: 20 minutes
Cooking Time: 6 to 8 hours
Serving: 4

Ingredients:

- 1 large sweet potato, peeled and chopped
- 5 cups water
- 2 cups baby carrots
- 2 cups chopped celery
- 1 yellow onion, chopped
- 1/8 teaspoon salt
- 1/8 teaspoon freshly ground black pepper
- 2 cups frozen baby peas
- 4 tablespoons extra-virgin olive oil

Direction:

1. 1.Place the sweet potato in a large saucepan, cover with water, and bring to a boil on high heat. Boil for 10 minutes, then drain the potato and discard the water.
2. 2.In the slow cooker, combine the sweet potato, water, carrots, celery, onion, salt, and pepper and stir.

3. 3.Cover and cook on low for 6 to 8 hours, or until the vegetables are tender.
4. 4.Stir in the peas and cook on high for 10 minutes.
5. 5.To serve, ladle into bowls and top each with 1 tablespoon of olive oil.
6. Ingredient Tip: To give this stew an Italian flair, add 1 teaspoon of dried Italian seasoning when you stir in the peas and serve the soup with some grated Parmesan or Romano cheese.

Nutrition Per Serving Calories: 259; Total fat: 14g; Saturated fat: 2g; Sodium: 263mg; Phosphorus: 122mg; Potassium: 566mg; Carbohydrates: 19g; Fiber: 6g; Protein: 5g; Sugar: 8g

71. Spinach and Crab Soup

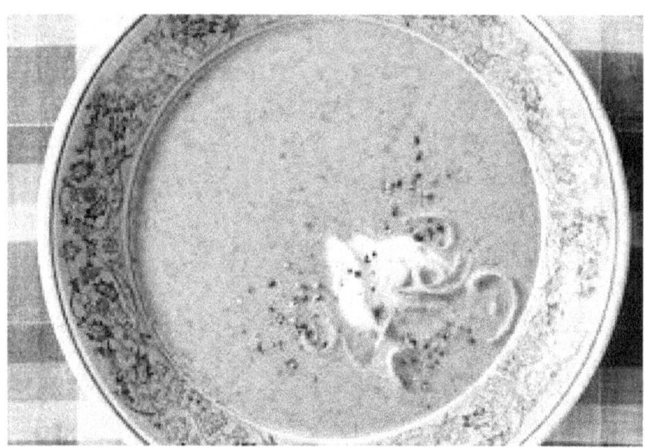

Preparation Time: 15 minutes
Cooking Time: 10 minutes
Serving: 4
Ingredients:

- 2 tablespoons extra-virgin olive oil
- 2 shallots, minced
- 8 ounces fresh lump crab meat, picked over
- 4 cups low-sodium vegetable broth

- 2 cups roughly chopped baby spinach leaves
- ½ teaspoon Old Bay Seasoning
- 1/8 teaspoon freshly ground black pepper

Direction:

1. 1.In a medium saucepan, heat the olive oil over medium heat. Cook the shallots for about 3 minutes, stirring, until tender.
2. 2.Add the crab meat and cook for 1 minute. Add the vegetable broth and bring to a simmer. Reduce the heat to low.
3. 3.Add the spinach leaves, Old Bay Seasoning mix, and pepper. Simmer until the spinach is wilted and the soup is hot. Serve.
4. Ingredient Tip: You could use other greens in place of the spinach. Try baby arugula leaves, frisée, or kale that has been torn into pieces.

Nutrition Per Serving Calories: 138; Total fat: 7g; Saturated fat: 1g; Sodium: 408mg; Phosphorus: 160mg; Potassium: 345mg; Carbohydrates: 6g; Fiber: 1g; Protein: 12g; Sugar: 3g

72.   Curried Lentil Soup

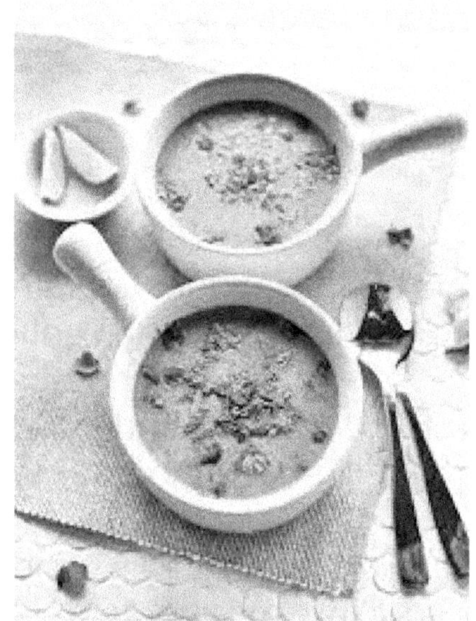

Preparation Time: 15 minutes
Cooking Time: 30 minutes
Serving: 4
Ingredients:

- ½ cup green lentils, sorted
- 2 tablespoons extra-virgin olive oil
- 1 yellow onion, chopped
- 1 tablespoon curry powder
- 4 cups low-sodium vegetable broth
- 2 large carrots, peeled and sliced
- 1/8 teaspoon salt
- 1/8 teaspoon freshly ground black pepper

Direction:

1. 1.In a medium saucepan, combine the lentils and the amount of water on the lentil package's instructions. Bring to a boil over medium heat. Reduce the heat to low and simmer for 10 minutes. Drain well, discarding the water.

2. 2.In a large saucepan, heat the olive oil over medium heat. Add the onion and curry powder and cook for about 3 minutes, stirring until the onion is tender.
3. 3.Add the lentils, broth, carrots, salt, and pepper and bring to a simmer. Simmer for 20 minutes or until the carrots and lentils are tender. Serve.
4. Increase Protein Tip: To make this a high-protein recipe, top each serving with 2 tablespoons of nonfat plain Greek yogurt. The protein content will increase to 11g per serving.

Nutrition Per Serving Calories: 186; Total fat: 8g; Saturated fat: 1g; Sodium: 240mg; Phosphorus: 101mg; Potassium: 379mg; Carbohydrates: 24g; Fiber: 5g; Protein: 7g; Sugar: 5g

73.   Simple Chicken and Rice Soup

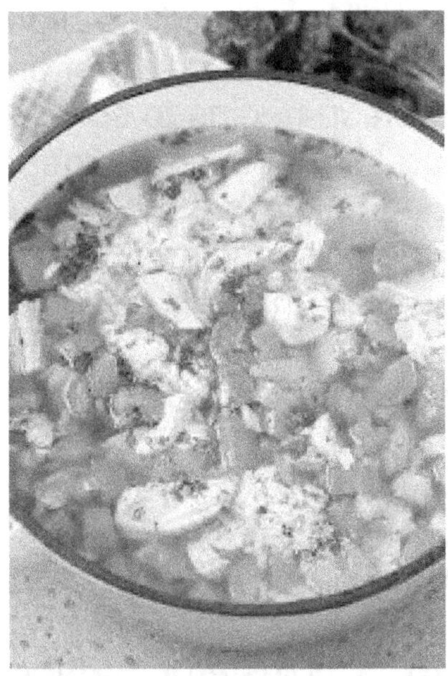

Preparation time: 10 minutes
Cooking time: 15 minutes
Servings: 4
Ingredients

- 1 tablespoon extra-virgin olive oil
- ½ sweet onion, chopped
- 2 celery stalks, chopped
- 2 carrots, chopped
- 8 ounces chicken breast, diced
- 4 cups simple chicken broth or low-sodium store-bought chicken stock
- ¼ teaspoon dried thyme leaves
- 1 cup cooked rice
- Juice of 1 lime
- Freshly ground black pepper
- 2 tablespoons chopped parsley leaves, for garnish

Directions:

1. In a medium stockpot, heat the olive oil over medium-high heat. Add the onion, celery, and carrots, and cook, often stirring for about 5 minutes until the onion begins to soften.
2. Add the chicken breast and continue stirring until the meat is just browned but not cooked through. Add the broth and thyme, and bring to a boil. Reduce the heat and simmer for 10 minutes, until the chicken is cooked through and the vegetables are tender.
3. Add the rice and lime juice. Season with pepper. Serve, garnished with parsley leaves.
4. Lower sodium tip: Choosing the simple chicken broth over the store-bought variety will allow you to control the amount of sodium in the finished product.

Nutrition: Calories: 176 Total fat: 11g Cholesterol: 26mg Carbohydrates: 17g Fiber: 3g Protein: 7g Phosphorus: 225mg Potassium: 357mg Sodium: 128mg

74.   Chicken Pho

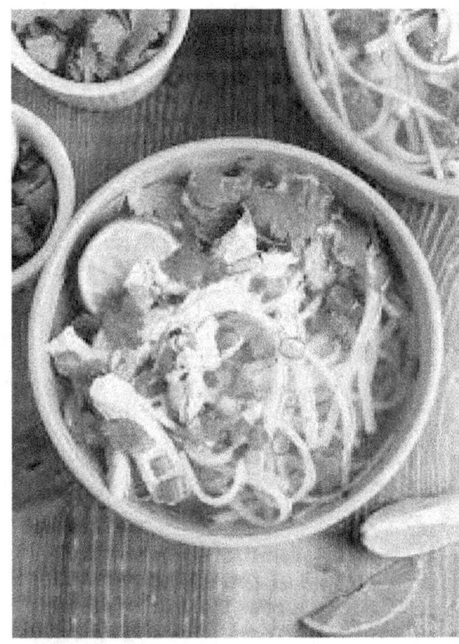

Preparation time: 10 minutes
Cooking time: 15 minutes
Servings: 4

Ingredients

- 5 cups simple chicken broth or low-sodium store-bought chicken stock
- 1-inch piece ginger, cut lengthwise into 2 or 3 strips
- 1 cup cooked chicken breast, diced
- Several fresh Thai basil sprigs
- 1 cup mung bean sprouts
- 1 lime, cut into wedges
- 1 jalapeño pepper, stemmed, seeded, and thinly sliced
- 1 (16-ounce) package dried rice vermicelli noodles, cooked according to package Directions
- 4 tablespoons (¼ cup) sliced scallions
- 4 tablespoons (¼ cup) chopped cilantro leaves

Directions

1. In a medium stockpot over medium-high heat, add the broth and ginger, and bring to a simmer. Add the chicken and simmer for 5 minutes. Remove the ginger from the pot and discard it.
2. On a plate, arrange the Thai basil, bean sprouts, lime wedges, and jalapeño slices.
3. Distribute the noodles among four bowls. Add 1¼ cups of broth to each bowl. Top with 1 tablespoon each of the scallions and cilantro. Serve immediately alongside the plate of garnishes.

Substitution tip: If you can't find fresh Thai basil near you, you can substitute regular basil, available in the fresh herb section of your grocery store.

Nutrition: Calories: 176 Total fat: 31g Cholesterol: 26mg Carbohydrates: 17g Fiber: 3g Protein: 7g Phosphorus: 225mg Potassium: 527mg Sodium: 138mg

75. Turkey Burger Soup

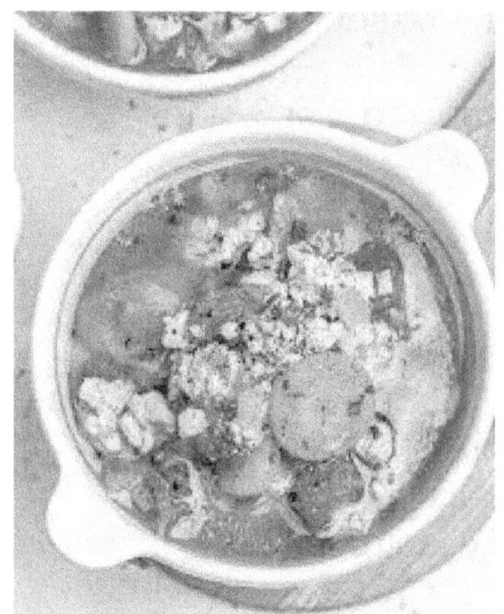

Preparation time: 10 minutes

Cooking time: 25 minutes
Servings: 4
Ingredients

- 2 tablespoons extra-virgin olive oil
- 1-pound ground turkey breast
- ½ sweet onion, chopped
- 3 garlic cloves, minced
- Freshly ground black pepper
- 1 (16-ounce) can low-sodium diced tomatoes, drained
- 4 cups simple chicken broth or low-sodium store-bought chicken stock
- 1 cup sliced carrots
- 1 cup sliced celery
- 1 tablespoon chopped fresh basil
- 1 tablespoon chopped fresh oregano
- 1 tablespoon chopped fresh thyme

Directions

1. In a medium stockpot over medium-high heat, heat the olive oil. Add the turkey, onion, and garlic. Cook and stir until the turkey is browned. Season with pepper.
2. Add the drained tomatoes, broth, carrots, celery, basil, oregano, and thyme. Reduce the heat to low, and simmer for 20 minutes. Serve.

Substitution tip: If you don't have fresh basil, oregano, or thyme, use dried instead. Substitute 1 teaspoon of dried herbs for each tablespoon of fresh.
Nutrition: Calories: 186 Fat: 11g Cholesterol: 26mg Carbohydrates: 17g Fiber: 3g Protein: 7g
Phosphorus: 115mg Potassium: 257mg Sodium: 128mg

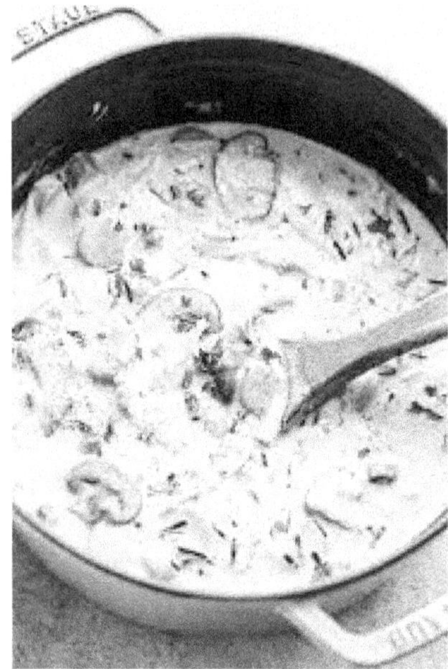

Preparation time: 15 minutes
Cooking time: 2–3 hours
Servings: 6

Ingredients

- ½ cup onion, chopped
- ½ cup red bell pepper, chopped
- ½ cup carrots, chopped
- 2 garlic cloves, minced
- 2 cup cooked turkey, shredded
- 5 cup chicken broth (see recipe)
- ½ cup quick-cooking wild rice, uncooked
- 1 tablespoon olive oil
- 1 cup mushrooms, sliced
- 2 bay leaves
- ¼ tablespoon Mrs. Dash® Original salt-free herb seasoning blend
- 1 tablespoon dried thyme

- ½ tablespoon low sodium salt
- ¼ tablespoon black pepper

Directions

1. Cook rice in a saucepan with 1–2 cups of broth. Set aside.
2. Heat the oil in a skillet and sauté the onion, bell pepper, carrots, and garlic until soft. Add to a 4 to 6-quart slow cooker.
3. Add the remaining ingredients to the slow cooker except for the rice and mushrooms.
4. Cover and cook for 2–3 hours on low.
5. Add the mushrooms and rice and cook for a further 15 minutes.
6. Remove the bay leaves and serve.

Nutrition: Calories: 136 Fat: 11g Cholesterol: 26mg Carbohydrates: 15g Fiber: 3g Protein: 5g Phosphorus: 145mg Potassium: 537mg Sodium: 128mg

## 77.	Green Chili Stew

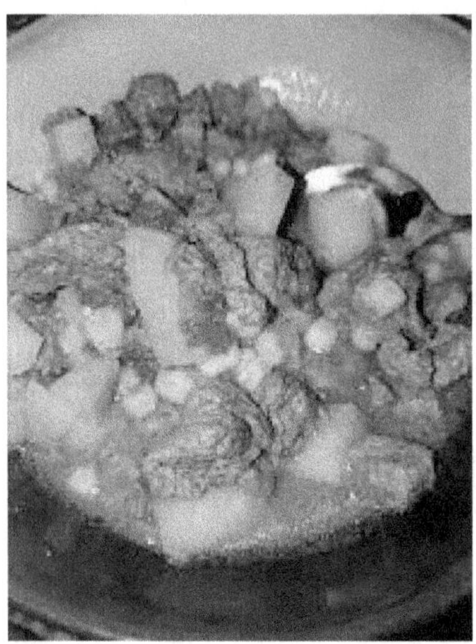

Preparation time: 20 minutes
Cooking time: 10 hours
Servings: 6

Ingredients

- ½ cup all-purpose flour
- 1 tablespoon garlic powder
- 1 tablespoon black pepper
- 1lb lean boneless pork chops, cut into 1-inch cubes
- 1 tablespoon olive oil
- 1 (8-ounces) can of green chili peppers, drained well and chopped
- 1 garlic clove, minced
- 2 cup chicken broth (see recipe)
- 6 flour tortillas, burrito size
- ¾ cup iceberg lettuce, shredded
- ¼ cup cilantro, finely chopped
- 6 tablespoon sour cream

Directions

1. Place the flour, garlic powder, and black pepper into a ziploc bag.
2. Add the pork and coat well.
3. Heat the oil in a skillet and brown the pork.
4. Add the pork to a 4-quart slow cooker along with the broth, peppers, and garlic.
5. Cover and cook for 10 hours on low.
6. Place lettuce on a tortilla, top with stew, and roll up burrito style.
7. Top with sour cream and cilantro.

Nutrition: Calories: 126 Fat: 11g Cholesterol: 26mg Carbohydrates: 17g Fiber: 3g Protein: 7g Phosphorus: 155mg Potassium: 357mg Sodium: 188mg

78. Golden Chickpea And Vegetable Soup

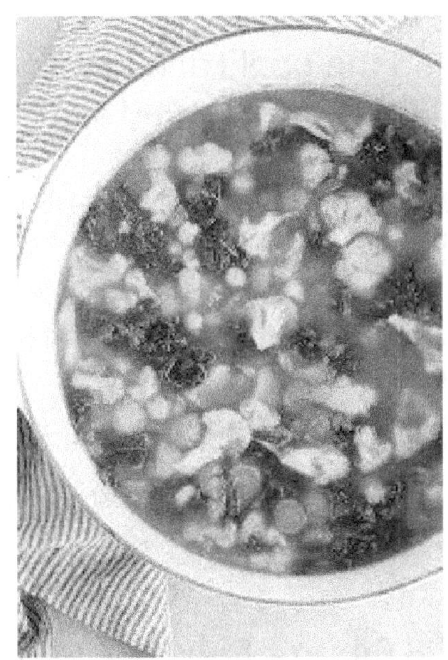

Preparation Time: 15 minutes
Cooking Time: 20 minutes
Servings: 6

Ingredients:

- 1 tbsp. Grated ginger
- 1 cup diced carrots
- 2 tsp. Coconut oil
- 2 tbsp. Curry powder
- 2 cups Cauliflower florets
- 2 cloves minced garlic
- 1 cup cooked chickpeas
- 1 ½ cup Diced celery
- 1 ½ cup Sliced leeks
- 4 cups Bone broth
- 2 tbsp. Minced organic parsley
- 1 cup Torn curly kale leaves

Directions:

1. Warm the coconut oil in a pot and add the garlic and ginger. Sauté for a minute before adding the turmeric and curry powder and sautéing for another minute.
2. Throw in celery, leeks, carrots, and cauliflower, constantly stirring for about a minute.
3. Add the bone broth and chickpeas. Cover the pot and leave to boil. Lower the heat and let it simmer for at least 15 minutes.
4. Turn off heat and add parsley and kale, leaving the heat to cook the leaves.
5. Sprinkle salt and pepper.
6. Serve.

Nutrition: Calories: 142 kcal Protein: 8.64 g Fat: 4.79 g Carbohydrates: 17.57 g

79. Spring Pea Soup

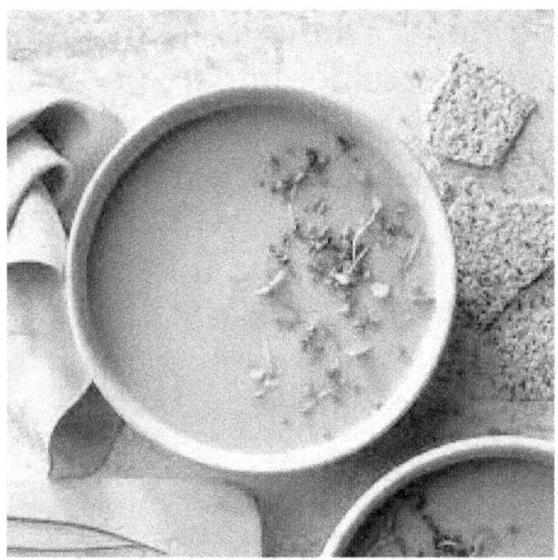

Preparation Time: 5 minutes
Cooking Time: 15 minutes
Servings: 6
Ingredients:

- 2 tbsp. Coconut oil
- 700 g. Fresh peas
- 1 medium Chopped onion
- Chopped mint leaves
- 1-liter Vegetable stock
- Chopped flat-leaf parsley
- Fresh lemon juice
- ½ tsp. ground cumin
- 2 tsp. Celtic sea salt
- Toasted sunflower seeds
- Grated nutmeg
- ½ tsp. Black pepper powder

Directions:

1. Warm the coconut oil in a pan set over medium heat.
2. Stir in onions and stir fry for about 5 minutes.

3. Put in the stock and raise the heat. Throw in fresh peas and cook for 5 minutes. If you're using frozen peas, it should take half the time.
4. Pour in the lemon juice, salt, pepper, herbs, and spices. Stirring constantly
5. Turn off the heat and let it cool before running it through a food processor to whatever consistency you like.
6. Serve with sunflower seed sprinkles and mint or parsley leaves.
7. Enjoy!

Nutrition: Calories: 115 kcal Protein: 5 g Fat: 5.91 g Carbohydrates: 11.8 g

80. Tuna macaroni salad

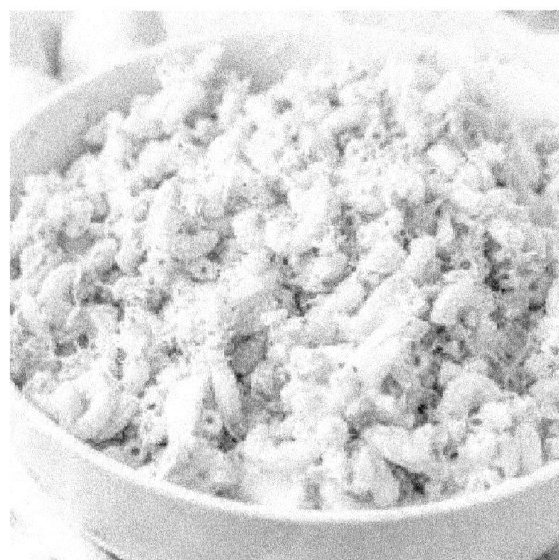

Preparation time: 5 minutes
Cooking time: 25 minutes
Servings: 10 servings
Ingredients:

- 1 1/2 cups Uncooked Macaroni
- 1 170g Can of tuna in water
- 1/4 cup Mayonnaise
- 2 medium celery stalks, diced
- 1 Tbsp. Lemon Pepper Seasoning

Directions:

1. Cook the pasta and let it cool in the refrigerator.
2. Drain the tuna in a colander and rinse it with cold water.
3. Add the tuna and celery once the macaroni has cooled.
4. Stir in mayonnaise and sprinkle with lemon seasoning. Mix well. Serve cold.

Nutrition: Power: 136 g, Protein: 8.0 g, Carbohydrates: 18 g, fibbers: 0.8 g, Fat: 3.6 g, Sodium: 75 mg, Potassium: 124 mg, Phosphorus: 90 mg

81. Fruity zucchini salad

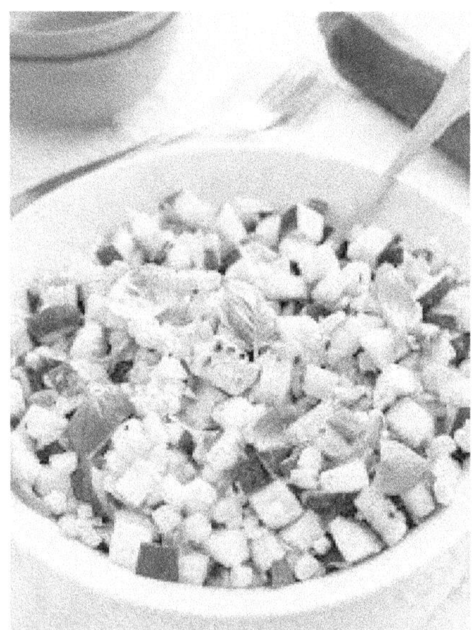

Preparation time: 5 minutes
Cooking time: 5 minutes
Servings: 4 servings
Ingredients:

- 400g zucchini
- 1 small onion
- 4 tbsp. olive oil
- 100g pineapple preserve, drained
- Salt, paprika
- thyme

Directions:

1. Dice the onions and sauté in the oil until translucent.

2. Cut the zucchini into slices and add. Season with salt, paprika, and thyme.
3. Let cool and mix with the cut pineapple.

Nutrition: Energy: 150kcal, Protein: 2g, Fat: 10g, Carbohydrates: 10g, Dietary fibbers: 2g, Potassium: 220mg, Calcium: 38mg, Phosphate: 24mg

82.   Hawaiian Chicken Salad

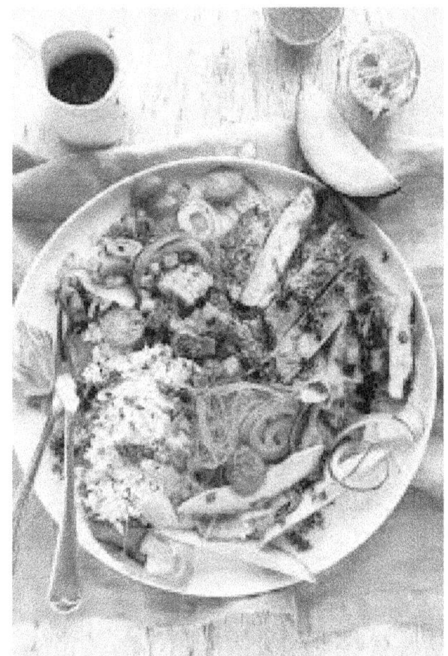

Preparation time: 5 minutes
Cooking time: 30 minutes
Servings: 4
Ingredients:

- 1 1/2 cups of chicken breast, cooked, chopped
- 1 cup pineapple chunks
- 1 1/4 cups lettuce iceberg, shredded
- 1/2 cup celery, diced
- 1/2 cup mayonnaise

- 1/8 tsp (dash) Tabasco sauce
- 2 lemon juice
- 1/4 tsp black pepper

Directions:

1. Combine the cooked chicken, pineapple, lettuce, and celery in a medium bowl. Just set aside.
2. In a small bowl, make the dressing. Mix the mayonnaise, Tabasco sauce, pepper, and lemon juice.
3. Use the chicken mixture to add the dressing and stir until well mixed.

Nutrition: Power: 310 g, Protein: 16.8 g, Carbohydrates: 9.6 g, fibbers: 1.1 g, Fat: 23.1 g, Sodium: 200 mg, Potassium: 260 mg, Phosphorus: 134 mg

83. Chicken and asparagus salad with watercress

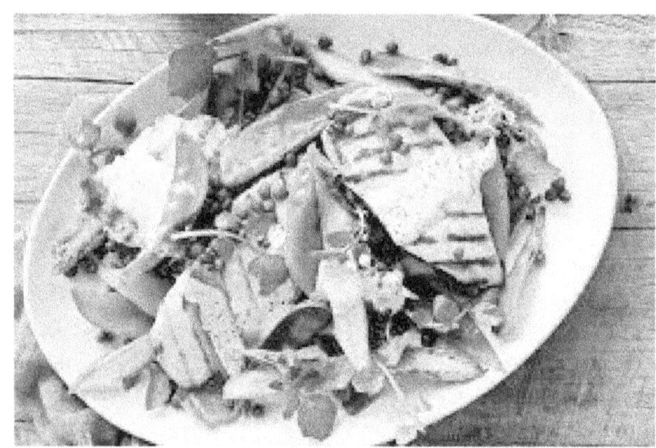

Preparation time: 5 minutes
Cooking time: 40 minutes
Serving: 4 servings
Ingredients:

- 100 g spring onions (0.5 bunch)

- 100 g green asparagus
- 600 g chicken breast fillet (4 chicken breast fillets)
- salt
- pepper
- 1 small lime
- 1 clove of garlic
- 6 tbsp. honey
- 1 tbsp. grainy mustard
- 5 tbsp. olive oil
- 100 g watercress

Directions:

1. The spring onions are cleaned and washed and then cut into thin rings.
2. The woody ends of the asparagus are cut off. Wash and pat the asparagus to dry. Halve the sticks and, with a peeler, cut the halves lengthwise into thin slices.
3. Wash the fillets of chicken, pat them dry with kitchen paper, and cut them into strips. With salt and pepper, season.
4. Trim the lime in half for the dressing and squeeze out the juice. Peel the garlic and dice it. Mix the mustard, 3 tablespoons of lime juice, and 3 tablespoons of oil with the honey. With salt and pepper, season.
5. In a large non-stick pan, heat the remaining oil and stir-fry the meat over high heat for about 5 minutes.
6. In a bowl, add the chicken, spring onions, and asparagus. Mix in the dressing and allow the salad too steep for 10 minutes or so.
7. Meanwhile, wash the cress and shake it dry. Pluck the leaves, chop coarsely as desired, and spread on dishes or bowls. Use salt and pepper to season the chicken salad and serve on the cress.

Nutrition: Calories 368 kcal (18%), Protein 37 g (38%), Fat 14 g (12%), Carbohydrates 22 g (15%), added sugar 17 g (68%), fibbers 2 g (7%)

84. Farmer's Salad

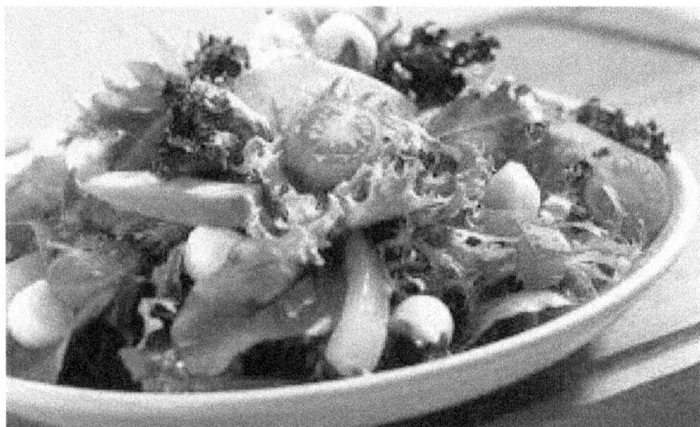

Preparation time: 5 minutes
Cooking time: 5 minutes
Servings: 2 servings
Ingredients:

- 60g mixed leaf salads
- 100g red pepper, diced
- 200g green beans
- 60g feta cheese
- 1 tbsp. wine vinegar
- 1 tbsp. diced onions
- Salt, pepper, sugar
- 2 tbsp. olive oil

Directions:

1. Mix vinegar with onions, oil, and spices and mix with the salad.

2. Cut the sheep's cheese into cubes and serve with the salad. It goes well with baguette or flatbread with herb butter.

Nutrition: Energy: 187kcal, Protein: 8g, Fat: 16g, Carbohydrates: 4g, Dietary fibers: 5g, Potassium: 396mg, Calcium: 188mg, Phosphate: 170mg

85. Couscous salad

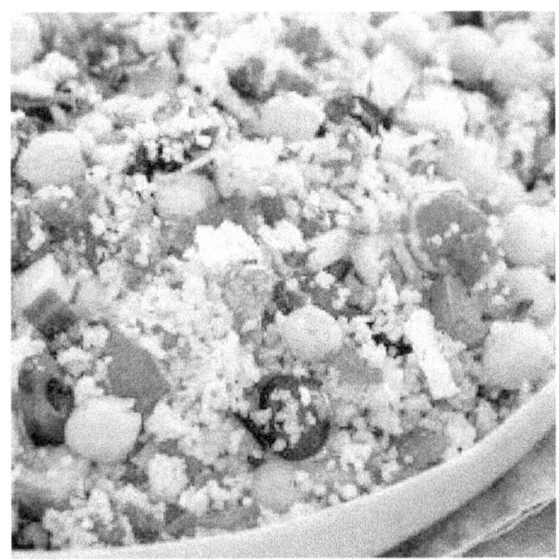

Preparation time: 5 minutes
Cooking time: 5 minutes
Servings: 5 servings
Ingredients:

- 3 cups of water
- 1/2 tsp. cinnamon tea
- 1/2 tsp. cumin tea
- 1 tsp. honey soup
- 2 tbsp. lemon juice
- 3 cups quick-cooking couscous
- 2 tbsp. tea of olive oil
- 1 green onion,

- Finely chopped 1 small carrot, finely diced
- 1/2 red pepper,
- Finely diced fresh coriander

Directions:

1. Stir in the water with the cinnamon, cumin, honey, and lemon juice and bring to a boil. Put the couscous in it, cover it, and remove it from the heat. To swell the couscous, stir with a fork. Add the vegetables, fresh herbs, and olive oil. It is possible to serve the salad warm or cold.

Nutrition: Energy: 190 g, Protein: 6 g, Carbohydrates: 38 g, fibbers: 2 g, Total Fat: 1 g, Sodium: 4 mg, Phosphorus: 82 mg, Potassium: 116 mg

86.   Tortellini salad

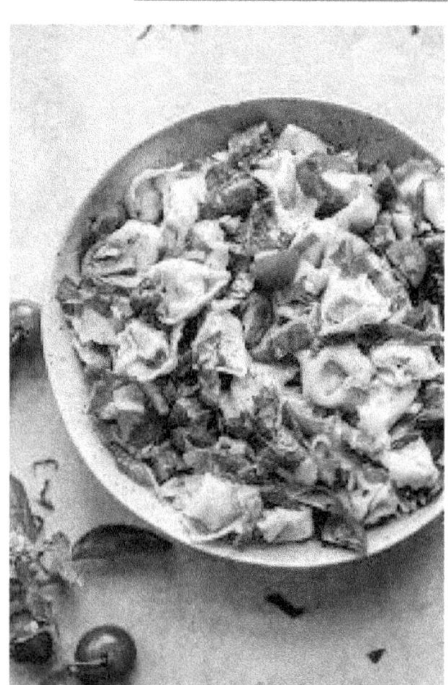

Preparation time: 5 minutes
Cooking time: 10 minutes
Servings: 4 servings

Ingredients:

- 200g tortellini with meat filling
- 100g red peppers
- 1 tomato
- 1 clove of garlic
- Salt pepper
- fresh basil, some leaves
- 3 tbsp. rapeseed oil
- 1 tbsp. white wine vinegar

Directions:

1. Cook the tortellini in salted water according to the instructions on the packet and drain.
2. Finely dice the pepper and garlic and sweat in the rapeseed oil. Add the vinegar and spices and pour over the tortellini. Cut the tomato into small pieces and mix in. mix with the fresh basil and season to taste.

Nutrition: Energy: 161kcal, Protein: 4g, Fat: 9g, Carbohydrates: 18g, Dietary fibbers: 3g, Potassium: 173mg, Phosphate: 80mg

87.   Cucumber Salad

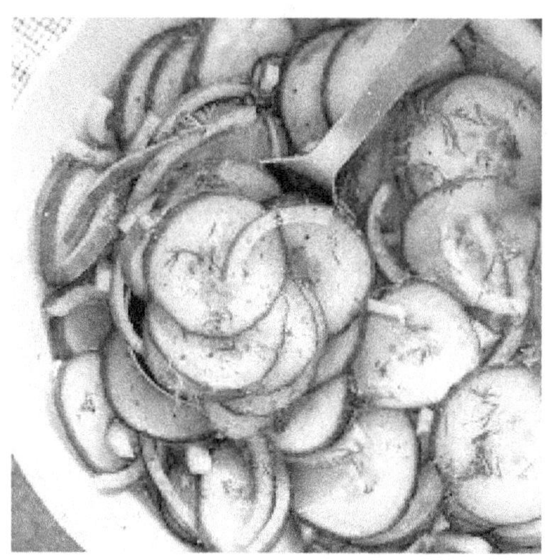

Preparation time:5 minutes
Cooking time: 5 minutes
Servings: 4
Ingredients:

- 1 tbsp. dried dill
- 1 onion
- ¼ cup water
- 1 cup vinegar
- 3 cucumbers
- ¾ cup white sugar

Direction:

1. In a bowl add all ingredients and mix well
2. Serve with dressing

Nutrition: Calories 49, Fat 0.1g, Sodium (Na) 341mg, Potassium (K) 171mg, Protein 0.8g, Carbs 11g, Phosphorus 24 mg

88.   Grated carrot salad with Lemon-Dijon vinaigrette

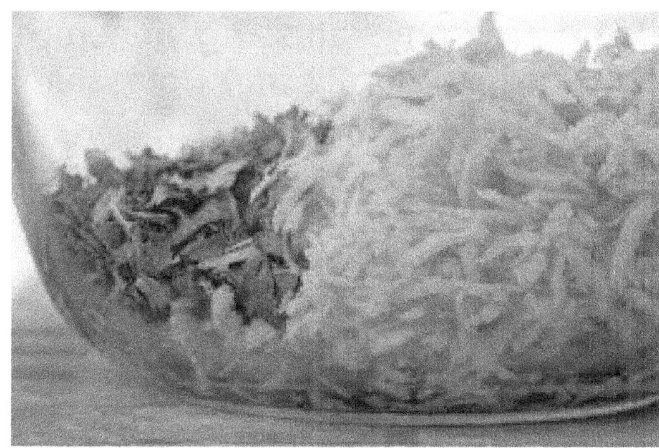

Preparation time: 15 minutes
Cooking time: 10 minutes
Servings: 8 servings
Ingredients:

- 9 small carrots (14 cm), peeled
- 2 tbsp. 1/2 teaspoon Dijon mustard
- 1 C. lemon juice
- 2 tbsp. extra virgin olive oil
- 1-2 tsp. honey (to taste)
- ¼ tsp. salt
- ¼ tsp. freshly ground pepper (to taste)
- 2 tbsp. chopped parsley
- 1 green onion, thinly sliced

Directions:

1. Grate the carrots in a food processor.
2. In a salad bowl, mix Dijon mustard, lemon juice, honey, olive oil, salt, and pepper. Add the carrots, fresh parsley, and green onions. Stir to coat well. Cover and refrigerate until ready to be serve.

Nutrition: Energy: 61 g, Proteins: 1 g, Carbohydrates: 7 g, fibbers: 1 g, Total Fat: 4 g, Sodium: 88 mg, Phosphorus: 22 mg, Potassium: 197 mg

89.   Broccoli-Cauliflower Salad

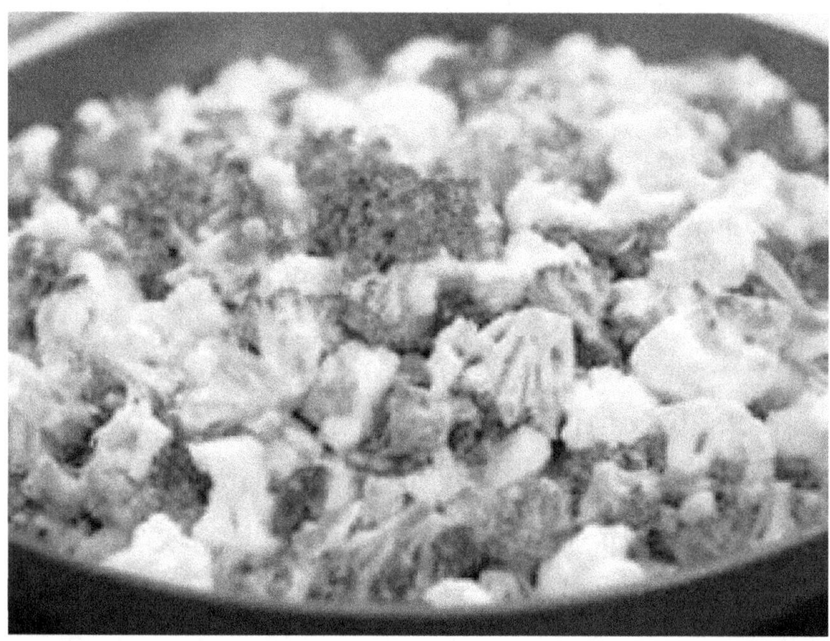

Preparation time:5minutes
Cooking time:5minutes
Servings: 4
Ingredients:

- 1 tbsp. wine vinegar
- 1 cup cauliflower florets
- ¼ cup white sugar
- 2 cups hard-cooked eggs
- 5 slices bacon
- 1 cup broccoli florets
- 1 cup cheddar cheese
- 1 cup mayonnaise

Direction:

1. In a bowl add all ingredients and mix well
2. Serve with dressing

Nutrition: Calories 89.8, Fat 4.5 g, Sodium (Na) 51.2 mg, Potassium (K) 257.6 mg, Carbs 11.5 g, Protein 3.0 g, Phosphorus 47 mg

90. Macaroni Salad

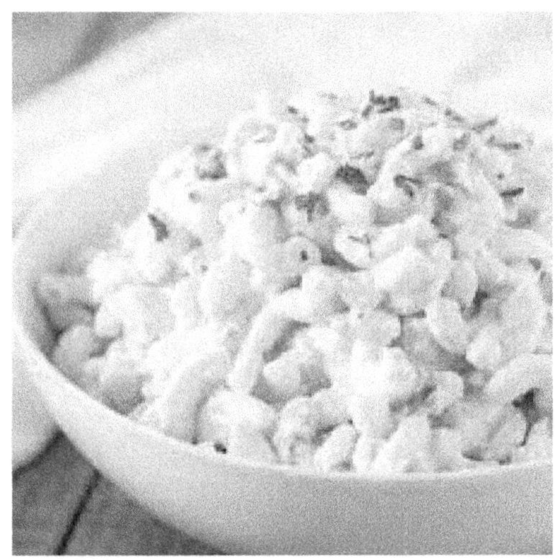

Preparation time:5minutes
Cooking time:5minutes
Servings: 4
Ingredients:

- ¼ tsp. celery seed
- 2 hard-boiled eggs
- 2 cups salad dressing
- 1 onion
- 2 tsps. white vinegar
- 2 stalks celery
- 2 cups cooked macaroni

- 1 red bell pepper
- 2 tbsps. mustard

Direction:

1. In a bowl add all ingredients and mix well
2. Serve with dressing

Nutrition: Calories 360, Fat 21g, Sodium (Na) 400mg, Carbs 36g, Protein 6g, Potassium (K) 68mg, Phosphorus 36 mg

91. Grapes Jicama Salad

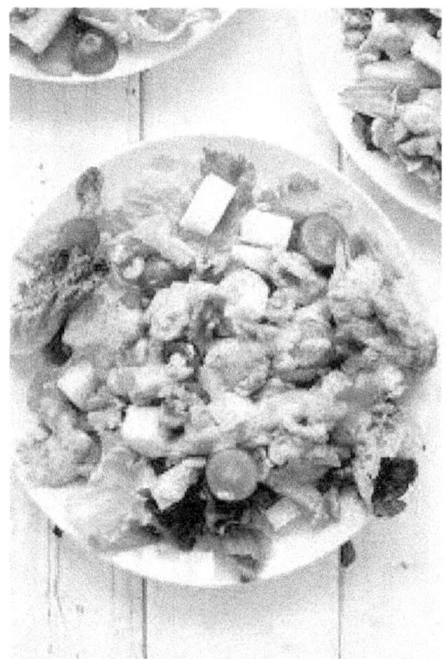

Preparation Time: 5 minutes
Cooking Time: 0 minutes
Servings: 2
Ingredients:

- 1 jicama, peeled and sliced
- 1 carrot, sliced
- 1/2 medium red onion, sliced

- 1 ¼ cup seedless grapes
- 1/3 cup fresh basil leaves
- 1 tablespoon apple cider vinegar
- 1 ½ tablespoon lemon juice
- 1 ½ tablespoon lime juice

Direction:

1. Put all the salad ingredients into a suitable salad bowl.
2. Toss them well and refrigerate for 1 hour.
3. Serve.

Nutrition: Calories 203 Total Fat 0.7g Sodium 44mg Protein 3.7g Calcium 79mg Phosphorous 141mg Potassium 429mg

92. Italian Cucumber Salad

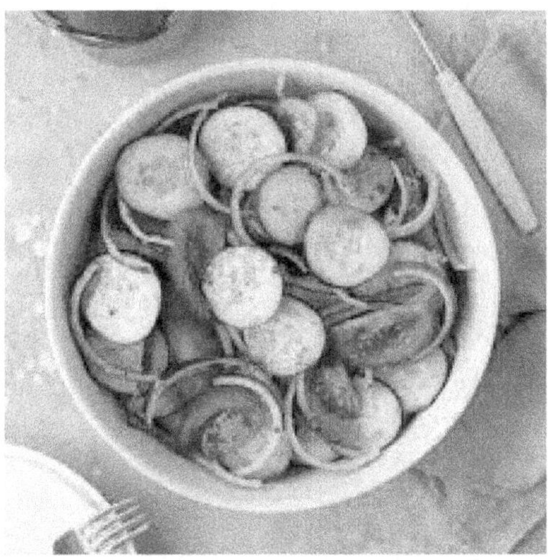

Preparation Time: 5 minutes
Cooking Time: 0 minutes
Servings: 2
Ingredients:

- 1/4 cup rice vinegar

- 1/8 teaspoon
- stevia
- 1/2 teaspoon olive oil
- 1/8 teaspoon black pepper
- 1/2 cucumber, sliced
- 1 cup carrots, sliced
- 2 tablespoons green onion, sliced
- 2 tablespoons red bell pepper, sliced
- 1/2 teaspoon Italian seasoning blend

Direction:

1. Put all the salad ingredients into a suitable salad bowl.
2. Toss them well and refrigerate for 1 hour.
3. Serve.

Nutrition: Calories 112 Total Fat 1.6g Cholesterol 0mg Sodium 43mg Protein 2.3g Phosphorous 198mg Potassium 529mg

93. Pear & Brie Salad

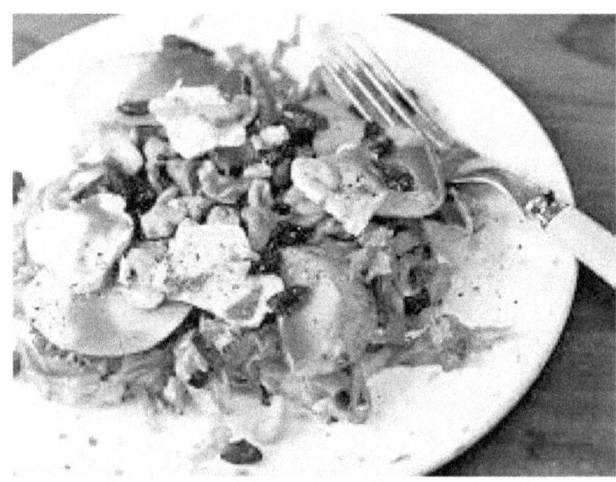

Preparation Time: 5 minutes
Cooking Time: 0 minutes
Servings: 4
Ingredients:

- 1 tablespoon olive oil
- 1 cup arugula
- ½ lemon
- ½ cup canned pears
- ¼ cucumber
- ¼ cup chopped brie

Direction:

1. Peel and dice the cucumber.
2. Dice the pear.
3. Wash the arugula.
4. Combine salad in a serving bowl and crumble the brie over the top.
5. Whisk the olive oil and lemon juice together.
6. Drizzle over the salad.
7. Season with a little black pepper to taste and serve immediately.

Nutrition: Calories 54, Protein 1 g, Carbs 12 g, Fat 7 g, Sodium 57mg, Potassium 115 mg, Phosphorus 67 mg

94. Caesar Salad

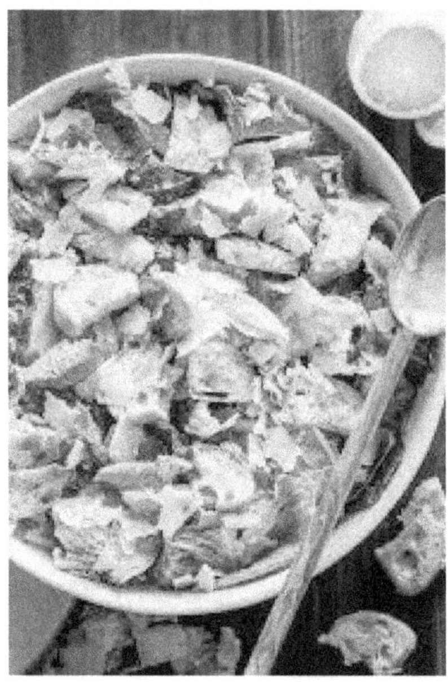

Preparation Time:5minutes
Cooking Time:5minutes
Servings: 4
Ingredients:

- 1 head romaine lettuce
- ¼ cup mayonnaise
- 1 tablespoon lemon juice
- 4 anchovy fillets
- 1 teaspoon Worcestershire sauce
- Black pepper
- 5 garlic cloves
- 4 tablespoons. Parmesan cheese
- 1 teaspoon mustard

Direction:

1. In a bowl mix all ingredients and mix well
2. Serve with dressing

Nutrition: Calories 44, Fat 2.1 g, Sodium 83 mg, Potassium 216 mg, Carbs 4.3 g, Protein 3.2 g, Phosphorus 45.6mg Calcium 19mg, Potassium 27mg Sodium: 121 mg

95.   Thai Cucumber Salad

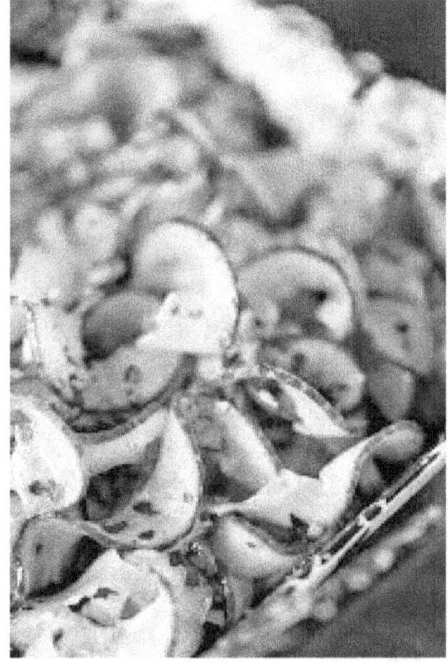

Preparation Time:5minutes
Cooking Time:5minutes
Servings: 2
Ingredients:

- ¼ cup chopped peanuts
- ¼ cup white sugar
- ½ cup cilantro
- ¼ cup rice wine vinegar
- 3 cucumbers
- 2 jalapeno peppers

Direction:

1. Add all ingredients in a small basin and combine well

2.	Serve with dressing

Nutrition: Calories 20, Fat 0g, Sodium 85mg, Carbs 5g, Protein 1g, Potassium 190.4 mg, Phosphorus 46.8mg

## 96.	Barb's Asian Slaw

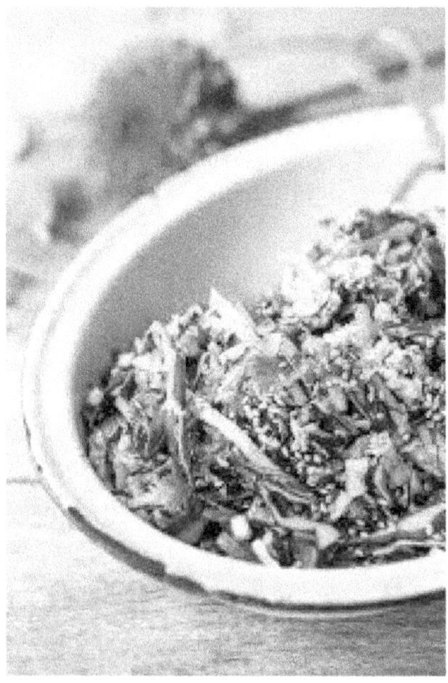

Preparation Time: 5 minutes
Cooking Time: 5 minutes
Servings: 2
Ingredients:

- 1 cabbage head, shredded
- 4 chopped green onions
- ½ cup slivered or sliced almonds

Dressing:

- ½ cup olive oil
- ¼ cup tamari or soy sauce
- 1 tablespoon honey or maple syrup

- 1 tablespoon baking stevia

Directions:

1. Heat up dressing ingredients in a saucepan on the stove until thoroughly mixed.
2. Mix all ingredients when you are ready to serve.

Nutrition: Calories: 205 Protein: 27g Carbohydrate: 12g Fat: 10 g Calcium 29mg, Phosphorous 76mg, Potassium 27mg Sodium: 111 mg

97.   Green Bean and Potato Salad

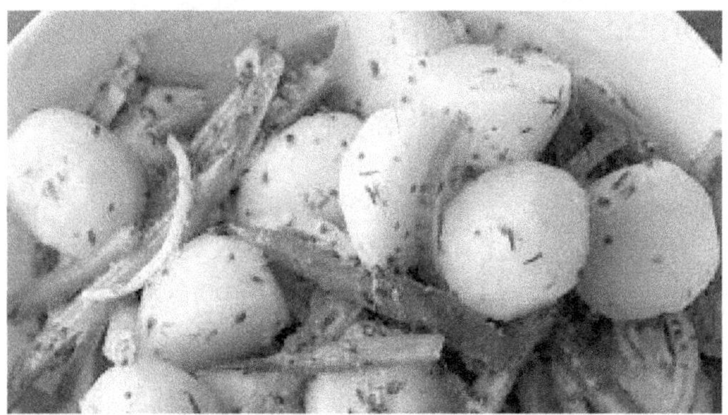

Preparation Time:5minutes
Cooking Time:5minutes
Servings: 4
Ingredients:

- ½ cup basil
- ¼ cup olive oil
- 1 tablespoon mustard
- ¾ lb. green beans
- 1 tablespoon lemon juice
- ½ cup balsamic vinegar
- 1 red onion

- 1 lb. red carrots
- 1 garlic clove

Direction:

1. Place carrots in a pot with water and bring to a boil for 15-18 minutes or until tender
2. Thrown in green beans after 5-6 minutes
3. Drain and cut into cubes
4. In a bowl add all ingredients and mix well
5. Serve with dressing

Nutrition: Calories 153.2, Fat 2.0 g, Sodium 77.6 mg, Potassium 759.0 mg, Carbs 29.0 g, Protein 6.9 g, Phosphorus 49 mg

98. Cucumber Couscous Salad

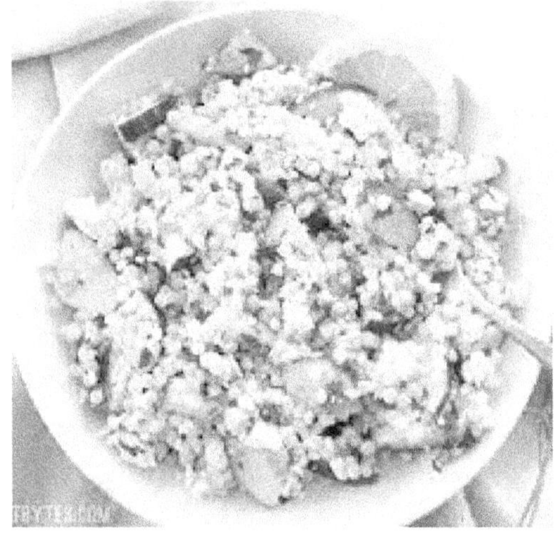

Preparation Time: 5 minutes
Cooking Time: 0 minutes
Servings: 4
Ingredients:

- 1 cucumber, sliced

- ½ cup red bell pepper, sliced
- ¼ cup sweet onion, sliced
- ¼ cup parsley, chopped
- ½ cup couscous, cooked
- 2 tablespoons olive oil
- 2 tablespoons rice vinegar
- 2 tablespoons feta cheese crumbled
- 1 ½ teaspoon dried basil
- 1/4 teaspoon black pepper

Direction:

1. Put all the salad ingredients into a suitable salad bowl.
2. Toss them well and refrigerate for 1 hour.
3. Serve.

Nutrition: Calories 202 Total Fat 9.8g Sodium 258mg Protein 6.2g Calcium 80mg Phosphorous 192mg Potassium 209mg

99.   <u>Pesto Chicken Mozzarella Salad</u>

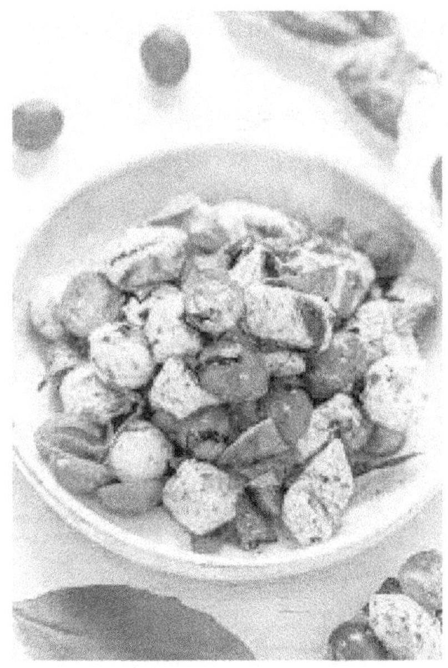

Preparation Time: 10 minutes
Cooking Time: 5 minutes
Servings: 4
Ingredients:

- 1 lb. cooked chicken, shredded
- 1/2 tbsp. fresh lemon juice
- 3 tbsp. pesto
- 1/2 cup yogurt
- 1/4 cup fresh basil, chopped
- 1/4 cup pine nuts
- 6 mozzarella balls, halved
- 1 cup cherry Red bell peppers, halved
- Pepper
- Salt

Directions:

1. In a small bowl, whisk together yogurt, lemon juice, pesto, pepper, and salt and set aside.
2. Add chicken, basil, pine nuts, mozzarella balls, and cherry Red bell peppers and mix well.
3. Pour dressing over salad and toss well and serve.

Nutrition: Calories 490 Fat 28.1 g Carbohydrates 5.9 g Sugar 4.4 g Protein 52.4 g Cholesterol 137 mg Phosphorus: 110mg Potassium: 117mg Sodium: 75mg

100. Skillet Chicken with Brussels Sprouts Mix

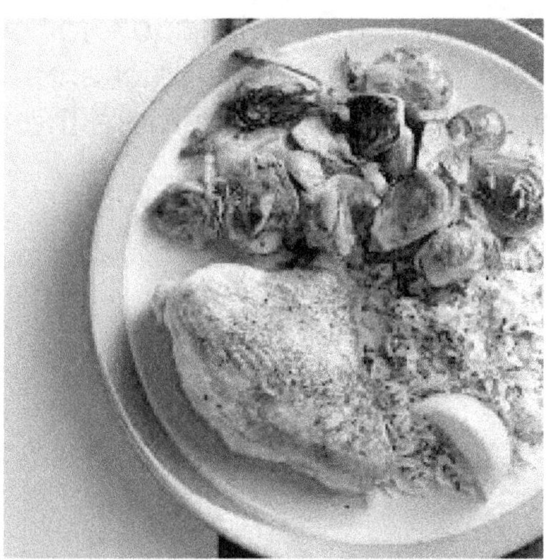

Preparation Time: 10 minutes
Cooking Time: 15 minutes
Servings: 4
Ingredients:

- 1½ pounds chicken thighs, skinless and boneless
- 1 tablespoon olive oil
- 2 teaspoons chopped thyme
- A pinch of salt and black pepper
- 12 ounces Brussel sprouts, shredded
- 1 apple, cored and sliced
- ½ red onion, sliced
- 1 garlic clove, minced
- 2 tablespoons balsamic vinegar
- ¼ cup walnuts, chopped

Directions:

1. Warm a pan with the oil over medium-high heat, then add the chicken thighs, season with salt, pepper, and thyme. Cook for 5 minutes on each side and transfer to a bowl. Heat the pan again over medium heat, add the onion, apple, sprouts, and garlic. Toss the mix and cook for 5 minutes. Add vinegar to the pan and return the chicken as well. Add the walnuts, toss, cook for 1-2 minutes more then divide between plates and serve.
2. Enjoy!

Nutrition: Calories: 211 Fat: 4 Fiber: 7 Carbs: 13 Protein: 8

101. Spicy Chipotle Chicken

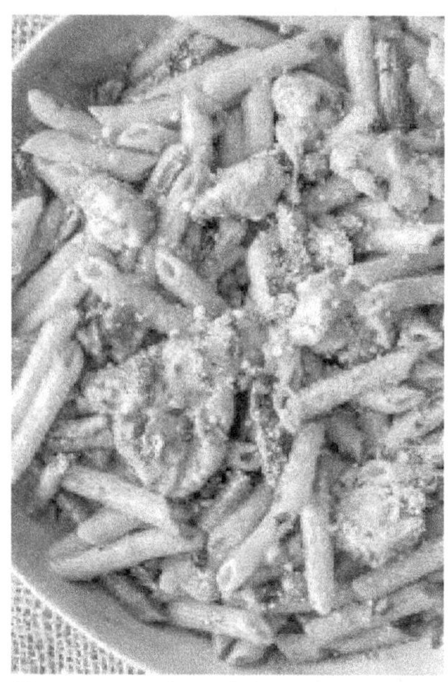

Preparation Time: 10 minutes
Cooking Time: 12 minutes
Servings: 4
Ingredients:

- 1-pound chicken breasts, skinless, boneless and cut into strips
- 1 teaspoon chili powder
- 1 teaspoon ground cumin
- A pinch of salt and black pepper
- 1 tablespoon olive oil
- 1 red bell pepper, sliced
- 1 cup halved mushrooms
- 1 yellow onion, chopped
- 3 garlic cloves, minced
- 1 tablespoon chopped chipotles in adobo
- 1½ tablespoons lime juice

Directions:

1. Warm a pan with the oil on medium-high heat and add the chicken. Mix and cook for 3-4 minutes. Add the chili powder, the cumin, salt, pepper, bell pepper, mushrooms, onion, garlic, chipotles, and lime juice. Mix and cook for 7 minutes more, divide into bowls and serve.
2. Enjoy!

Nutrition: Calories: 241 Fat: 4 Fiber: 7 Carbs: 14 Protein: 7

102. Chicken with Fennel

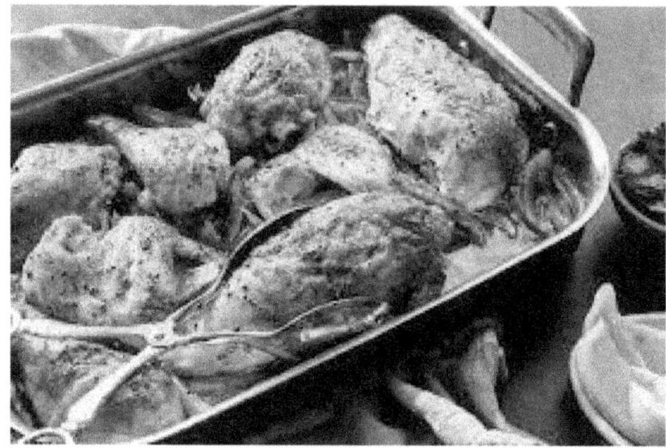

Preparation Time: 10 minutes
Cooking Time: 8 minutes
Servings: 4
Ingredients:

- 1 ¼ pounds chicken cutlets
- 1 ½ teaspoon smoked paprika
- A pinch of salt and black pepper
- 3 tablespoons olive oil
- 1 fennel bulb, sliced
- ¾ cup fennel fronds
- 1/3 cup red onion, sliced
- 1 almond, peeled, pitted and sliced
- 2 tablespoons lemon juice

Directions:

1. Warm a pan with 1 tbsp. Olive oil on medium-high heat temperature, then add the chicken, season with salt, pepper, and smoked paprika and cook for 4 minutes on each side. Divide between plates. In a bowl, mix the rest of the oil with the fennel, fennel fronds, onion, almond, and lemon juice. Toss the salad and place next to the chicken then serve.

2. Enjoy!

Nutrition: Calories: 288 Fat: 4 Fiber: 6 Carbs: 12 Protein: 7

103. Adobo Lime Chicken Mix

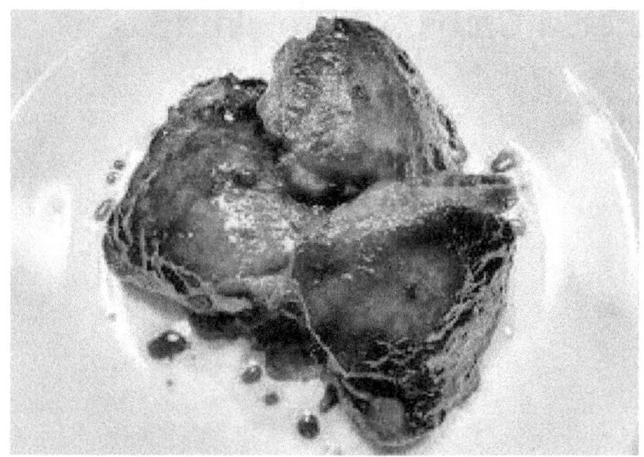

Preparation Time: 10 minutes
Cooking Time: 40 minutes
Servings: 6
Ingredients:

- 6 chicken thighs
- Salt and black pepper to the taste
- 1 tablespoon olive oil
- Zest of 1 lime
- 1½ teaspoons chipotle peppers in adobo sauce
- 1 cup sliced peach
- 1 tablespoon lime juice

Directions:

1. Warm a pan with the oil on medium-high heat and add the chicken thighs. Season with salt and pepper, then brown for 4 minutes on each side and bake in the oven at 375 degrees F for 20 minutes. In your food processor, mix the

peaches with the chipotle, lime zest, and lime juice, then blend and pour over the chicken. Bake for 10 minutes more, divide everything between plates and serve.

2. Enjoy!

Nutrition: Calories: 309 Fat: 6 Fiber: 4 Carbs: 16 Protein: 15

104. Cajun Chicken & Prawn

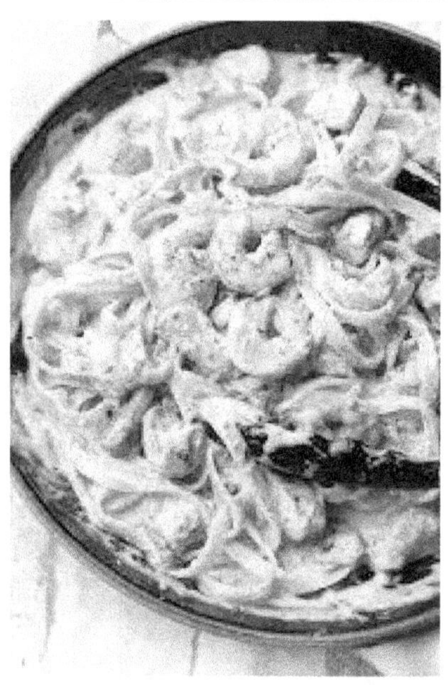

Preparation Time: 5 minutes
Cooking Time: 35 minutes
Servings: 2
Ingredients:

- 2 Free-range Skinless Chicken breast, chopped
- 1 Onion, chopped
- 1 Red pepper, chopped
- 2 Garlic cloves, crushed
- 10 Fresh or frozen prawn
- 1 tsp. Cayenne powder

- 1 tsp. Chili powder
- 1 tsp. Paprika
- 1/4 tsp. Chili powder
- 1 tsp. Dried oregano
- 1 tsp. Dried thyme
- 1 cup Brown or wholegrain rice
- 1 tbsp. Extra Virgin olive oil
- 1 can Bell pepper, chopped
- 2 cups Homemade chicken stock

Directions:

1. In a bowl, put all the spices and herbs then mix to form your Cajun spice mix.
2. Grab a large pan and add the olive oil, heating on medium heat.
3. Add the chicken and brown each side for around 4-5 minutes. Place to one side.
4. Add the onion to the pan and fry until soft.
5. Add the garlic, prawns, Cajun seasoning, and red pepper to the pan and cook for around 5 minutes or until prawns become opaque.
6. Add the white rice along with the chopped bell pepper, chicken, and chicken stock to the pan.
7. Cover the pan and allow to simmer for around 25 minutes or until the rice is soft.
8. Serve and enjoy!

Nutrition: Calories: 557 kcal Protein: 18.96 g Fat: 12.34 g Carbohydrates: 93.28 g

105. Healthy Turkey Gumbo

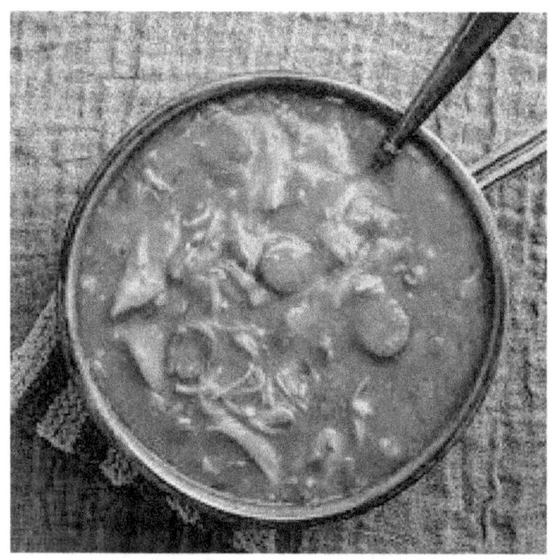

Preparation Time: 5 minutes
Cooking Time: 2 hours
Servings: 1
Ingredients:

- 1 Whole Turkey
- 1 Onion, quartered
- Stalk of Celery, chopped
- 3 Cloves garlic, chopped
- 1/2 cup Okra
- 1 can chopped bell pepper
- 1 tbsp. Extra virgin olive oils
- 1-2 Bay leaves
- Black pepper to taste

Directions:

1. Take the first four ingredients and add 2 cups of water in a stockpot, heating on a high heat until boiling.
2. Lower the heat and simmer for 45-50 minutes or until turkey is cooked through.
3. Remove the turkey and strain the broth.

4. Grab a skillet and then heat the oil on medium heat and brown the rest of the vegetables for 5-10 minutes.
5. Stir until tender, and then add to the broth.
6. Add the bell pepper and turkey meat to the broth and stir.
7. Add the bay leaves and continue to cook for an hour or until the sauce has thickened.
8. Season with black pepper and enjoy.

Nutrition: Calories: 261 kcal Protein: 11.72 g Fat: 12.91 g Carbohydrates: 28.33 g

106. Chinese-Mango Spiced Duck Breasts

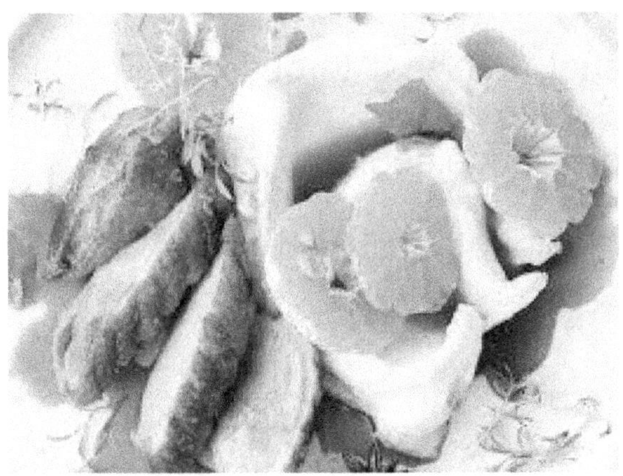

Preparation Time: 4 minutes
Cooking Time: 20 minutes
Servings: 2
Ingredients:

- 1 tsp. EXTRA Virgin olive oil
- 2 Duck breasts, skin removed
- 1 White onion, sliced
- 3 Cloves garlic, minced
- 2 tsp. Ginger, grated
- 1 tsp. Cinnamon
- 1 tsp. Cloves

- 1 Mango-Zest and Juice (Reserved the wedges)
- 2 Bok or Pak Choy plants leaves separated

Directions:

1. Slice the duck breasts into strips and add to a dry, hot pan, cooking for 5-7 minutes on each side or until cooked through to your liking.
2. Remove to one side.
3. Add olive oil to a clean pan and sauté the onions with the ginger, garlic, and the rest of the spices for 1 minute.
4. Put the juice and zest of the mango and continue to sauté for 3-5 minutes.
5. Add the duck and bok choi and heat through until wilted and duck is piping hot.
6. Serve and garnish with the mango segments.

Nutrition: Calories: 267 kcal Protein: 36.58 g Fat: 11.1 g Carbohydrates: 3.31 g

107. Super Sesame Chicken Noodles

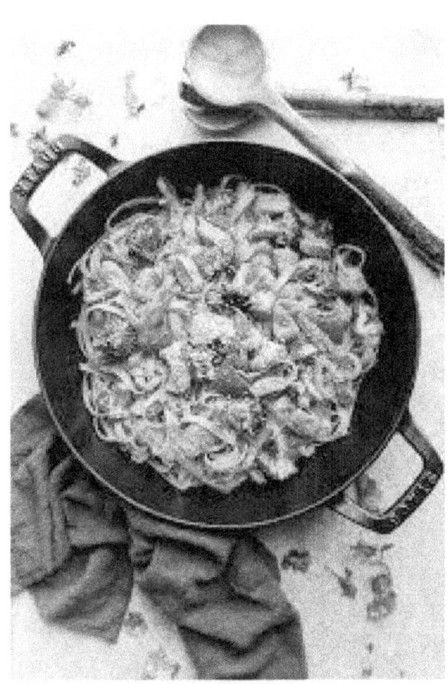

Preparation Time: 10 minutes
Cooking Time: 10 minutes
Servings: 2
Ingredients:

- 2 Free-range skinless chicken breasts, chopped
- 1 cup Rice/Buckwheat noodles such as Japanese Udon
- 1 Carrot, chopped
- 1/2 mango juiced
- 1 tsp. Sesame Seed
- 2 tsp. Coconut Oil
- 1 Thumb size piece of ginger, minced
- 1/2 cup Sugar snap peas

Directions:

1. Warm 1 tsp oil on medium heat in a skillet.
2. Sauté the chopped chicken breast for about 10-15 minutes or until cooked through.

3. While cooking the chicken, place the noodles, carrots, and peas in a pot of boiling water for about 5 minutes. Drain.
4. In a bowl, mix together the ginger, sesame seeds, 1 tsp oil, and mango juice to make your dressing.
5. Once the chicken is cooked and noodles are cooked and drained, add the chicken, noodles, carrots, and peas to the dressing and toss.
6. Serve warm or chilled.

Nutrition: Calories: 168 kcal Protein: 5.31 g Fat: 8.66 g Carbohydrates: 19.34 g

108. Lebanese Chicken Kebabs and Hummus

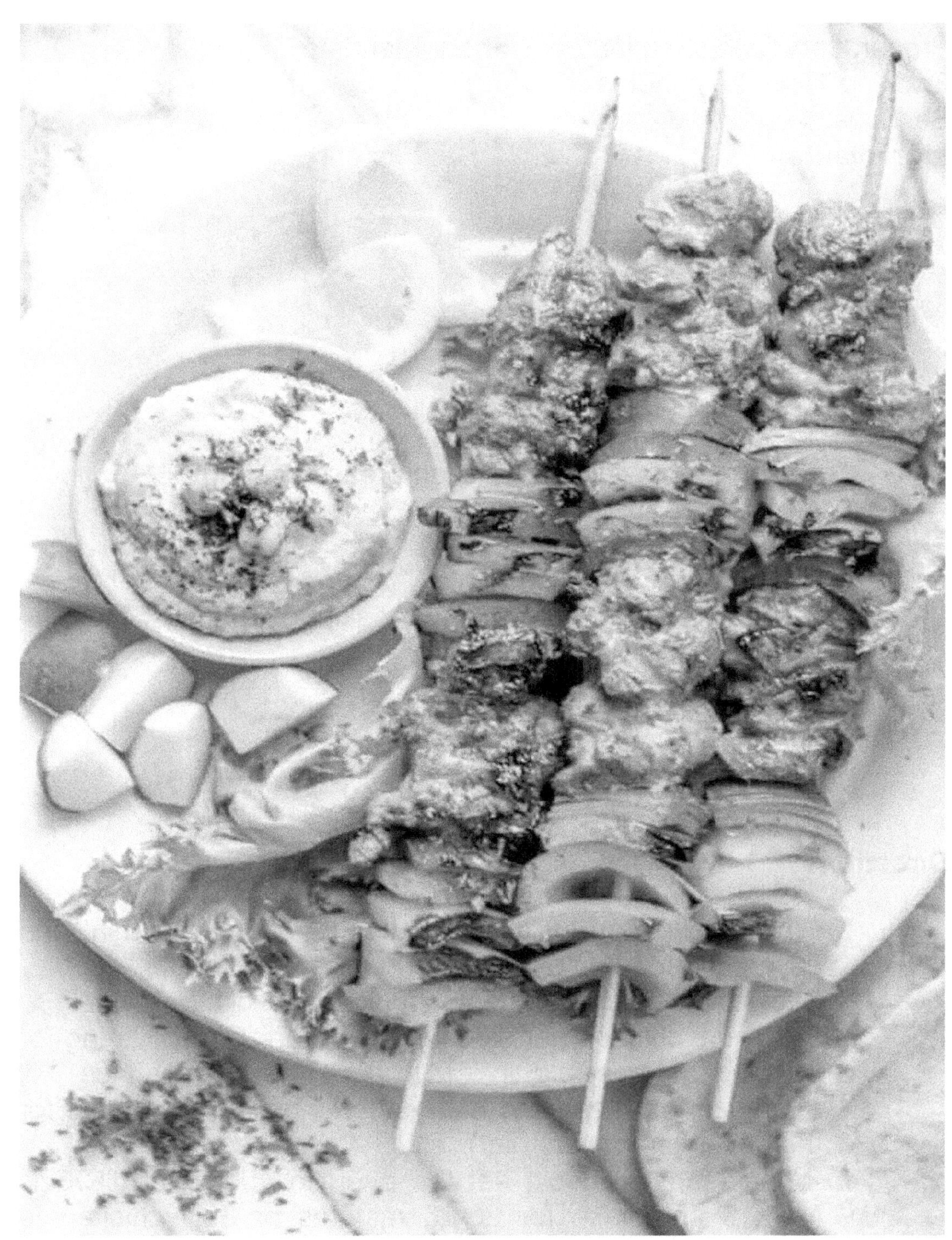

Preparation Time: 10 minutes + 1 hour marinate
Cooking Time: 35 minutes
Servings: 4

Ingredients:

- For the Chicken:
- 1 cup Lemon Juice
- 8 Garlic cloves, minced
- 1 tbsp. Thyme, finely chopped
- 1 tbsp. Paprika
- 2 tsp. ground cumin
- 1 tsp. Cayenne pepper
- 4 Free-range skinless chicken breasts, cubed
- 4 Metal kebabs skewers
- Lemon wedges to garnish
- For the Hummus:
- 1 can Chickpeas/ 1 cup dried (soaked overnight)
- 2 tbsp. Tahini paste
- 1 Lemon juice
- 1 tsp. Turmeric
- 1 tsp. Black pepper
- 2 tbsp. Olive oil

Directions:

1. Whisk the lemon juice, garlic, thyme, paprika, cumin, and cayenne pepper in a bowl.
2. Skewer the chicken cubes using kebab sticks (metal).
3. Baste the chicken per side with the marinade, covering for as long as possible in the fridge (the lemon juice will tenderize the meat and means it will be more suitable for the anti-inflammatory diet).
4. When ready to cook, set the oven to 400°F/200 °C/Gas Mark 6 and bake for 20-25 minutes or until chicken is

thoroughly cooked through.

5. Prepare the hummus by putting the ingredients to a blender and whizzing up until smooth. If it is a little thick and chunky, add a little water to loosen the mix.
6. Serve the chicken kebabs, garnished with the lemon wedges and the hummus on the side.

Nutrition: Calories: 576 kcal Protein: 61.66 g Fat: 18.55 g Carbohydrates: 42.07 g

109. Nutty Pesto Chicken Supreme

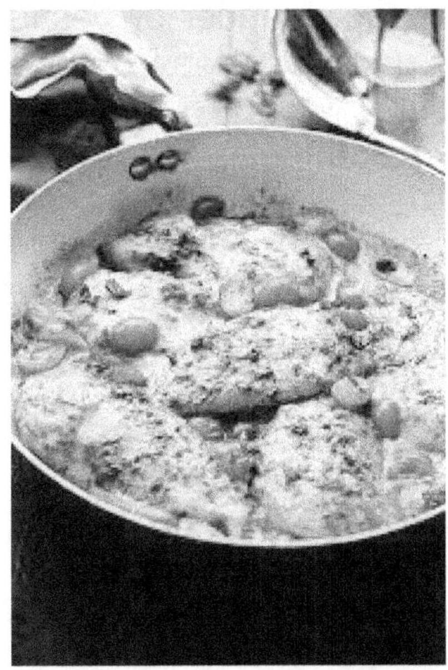

Preparation Time: 10 minutes
Cooking Time: 30 minutes
Servings: 2
Ingredients:

- 2 Free ranges skinless chicken/ turkey breasts
- 1 bunch of fresh basil
- 1/2 cup raw spinach

- 1 cup Crashed macadamias/almonds/walnuts or a combination
- 2 tbsp. Extra virgin olive oil
- 1/2 cup low-fat hard cheese (optional)

Directions:

1. Set the oven to 350°F.
2. Get the chicken breasts and use a meat pounder to 'thin' each breast into a 1cm thick escalope.
3. Reserve a handful of the nuts before adding the rest of the ingredients and a little black pepper to a blender or pestle and mortar and blend until smooth (you can leave this a little chunky for a rustic feel if you wish).
4. Add a little water if the pesto needs loosening.
5. Coat the chicken in the pesto.
6. Bake for at least 30 minutes in the oven, or until chicken is completely cooked through.
7. Top each chicken escalope with the remaining nuts and place under the broiler for 5 minutes for a crispy topping to complete.

Nutrition: Calories: 2539 kcal Protein: 444.61 g Fat: 71.66 g Carbohydrates: 5.99 g

110. Beef and Chili Stew

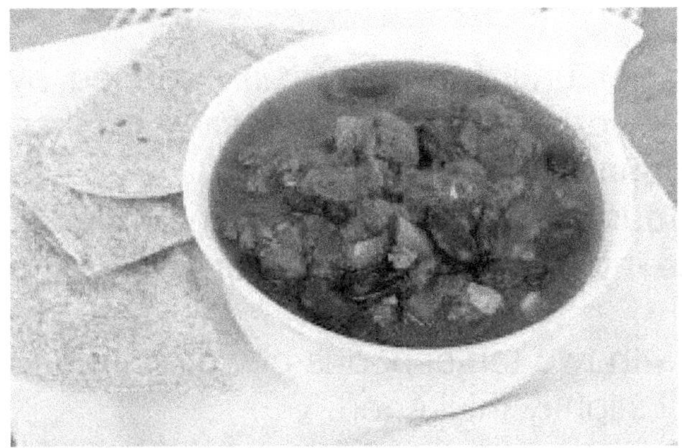

Preparation Time: 15 minutes
Cooking Time: 7 hours
Servings: 6
Ingredients:

- 1/2 medium red onion, sliced thinly
- 1/2 tablespoon vegetable oil
- 10ounce of flat-cut beef brisket, whole
- ½ cup low sodium stock
- ¾ cup of water
- ½ tablespoon honey
- ½ tablespoon chili powder
- ½ teaspoon smoked paprika
- ½ teaspoon dried thyme
- 1 teaspoon black pepper
- 1 tablespoon corn starch

Directions:

1. Throw the sliced onion into the slow cooker first. Add a splash of oil to a large hot skillet and briefly seal the beef on all sides.
2. Remove the beef, then place it in the slow cooker. Add the stock, water, honey, and spices to the same skillet you

cooked the beef meat.

3. Allow the juice to simmer until the volume is reduced by about half. Pour the juice over beef in the slow cooker. Cook on low within 7 hours.
4. Transfer the beef to your platter, shred it using two forks. Put the rest of the juice into a medium saucepan. Bring it to a simmer.
5. Whisk the cornstarch with two tablespoons of water. Add to the juice and cook until slightly thickened.
6. For a thicker sauce, simmer and reduce the juice a bit more before adding cornstarch. Put the sauce on the meat and serve.

Nutrition: Calories: 128 Protein: 13g Carbohydrates: 6g Fat: 6g Sodium: 228mg Potassium: 202mgPhosphorus: 119mg

111. Sticky Pulled Beef Open Sandwiches

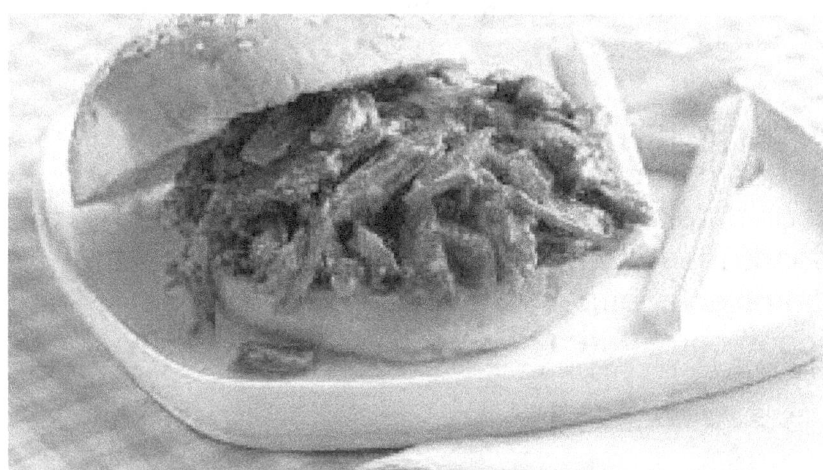

Preparation Time: 15 minutes
Cooking Time: 5 hours
Servings: 5
Ingredients:

- ½ cup of green onion, sliced
- 2 garlic cloves
- 2 tablespoons of fresh parsley
- 2 large carrots
- 7ounce of flat-cut beef brisket, whole
- 1 tablespoon of smoked paprika
- 1 teaspoon dried parsley
- 1 teaspoon of brown sugar
- ½ teaspoon of black pepper
- 2 tablespoon of olive oil
- ¼ cup of red wine
- 8 tablespoon of cider vinegar
- 3 cups of water
- 5 slices white bread
- 1 cup of arugula to garnish

Directions:

1. Finely chop the green onion, garlic, and fresh parsley. Grate the carrot. Put the beef in to roast in a slow cooker.
2. Add the chopped onion, garlic, and remaining ingredients, leaving the rolls, fresh parsley, and arugula to one side. Stir in the slow cooker to combine.
3. Cover and cook on low within 8 1/2 to 10 hours or on high for 4 to 5 hours until tender. Remove the meat from the slow cooker. Shred the meat using two forks.
4. Return the meat to the broth to keep it warm until ready to serve. Lightly toast the bread and top with shredded beef, arugula, fresh parsley, and ½ spoon of the broth. Serve.

Nutrition: Calories: 273 Protein: 15g Carbohydrates: 20g Fat: 11g Sodium: 308mg Potassium: 399mg Phosphorus: 159mg

112. Herby Beef Stroganoff and Fluffy Rice

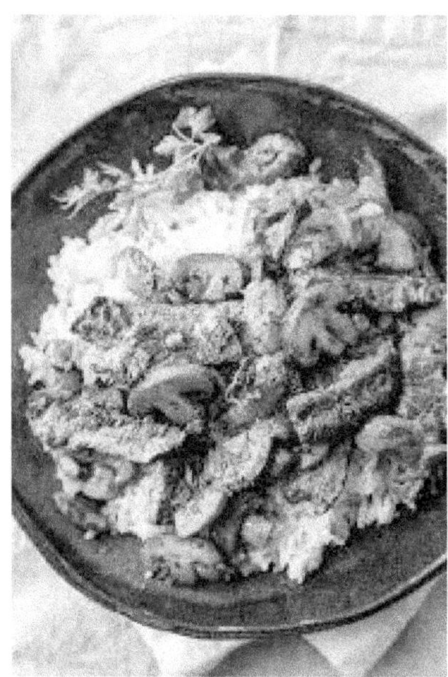

Preparation Time: 15 minutes
Cooking Time: 5 hours
Servings: 6

Ingredients:

- ½ cup onion
- 2 garlic cloves
- 9ounce of flat-cut beef brisket, cut into 1" cubes
- ½ cup of reduced-sodium beef stock
- 1/3 cup red wine
- ½ teaspoon dried oregano
- ¼ teaspoon freshly ground black pepper
- ½ teaspoon dried thyme
- ½ teaspoon of saffron
- ½ cup almond milk (unenriched)
- ¼ cup all-purpose flour
- 1 cup of water
- 2 ½ cups of white rice

Directions:

1. Dice the onion, then mince the garlic cloves. Mix the beef, stock, wine, onion, garlic, oregano, pepper, thyme, and saffron in your slow cooker.
2. Cover and cook on high within 4-5 hours. Combine the almond milk, flour, and water. Whisk together until smooth.
3. Add the flour mixture to the slow cooker. Cook for another 15 to 25 minutes until the stroganoff is thick.
4. Cook the rice using the package instructions, leaving out the salt. Drain off the excess water. Serve the stroganoff over the rice.

Nutrition: Calories: 241 Protein: 15g Carbohydrates: 29g Fat: 5g Sodium: 182mg Potassium: 206mg Phosphorus: 151mg

113. Chunky Beef and Potato Slow Roast

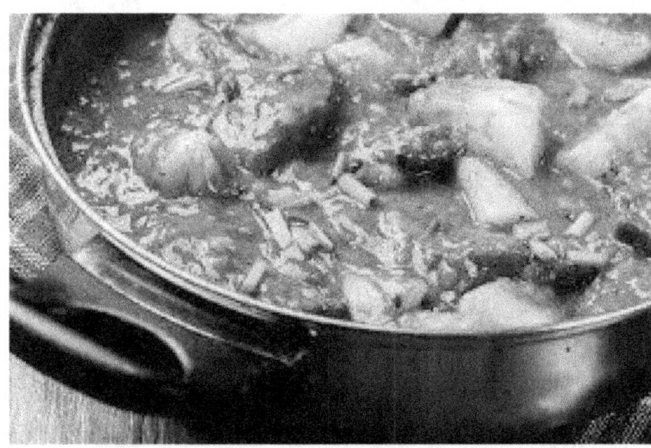

Preparation Time: 15 minutes
Cooking Time: 5-6 hours
Servings: 12
Ingredients:

- 3 cups of peeled carrots, chunked
- 1 cup of onion
- 2 garlic cloves, chopped
- 1 ¼ pound flat-cut beef brisket, fat trimmed

- 2 cups of water
- 1 teaspoon of chili powder
- 1 tablespoon of dried rosemary
- For the sauce:
- 1 tablespoon of freshly grated horseradish
- ½ cup of almond milk (unenriched)
- 1 tablespoon lemon juice (freshly squeezed)
- 1 garlic clove, minced
- A pinch of cayenne pepper

Directions:

1. Double boil the carrots to reduce their potassium content. Chop the onion and the garlic. Place the beef brisket in a slow cooker. Combine water, chopped garlic, chili powder, and rosemary.
2. Pour the mixture over the brisket. Cover and cook on high within 4-5 hours until the meat is very tender. Drain the carrots and add them to the slow cooker.
3. Adjust the heat to high and cook covered until the carrots are tender. Prepare the horseradish sauce by whisking together horseradish, almond milk, lemon juice, minced garlic, and cayenne pepper.
4. Cover and refrigerate. Serve your casserole with a dash of horseradish sauce on the side.

Nutrition: Calories: 199 Protein: 21gCarbohydrates: 12g Fat: 7g Sodium: 282mg Potassium: 317 Phosphorus: 191mg

114. Spiced Lamb Burgers

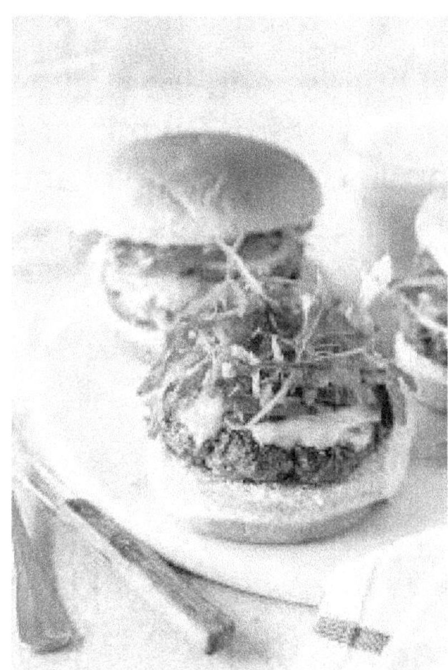

Preparation Time: 10 minutes
Cooking Time: 20 minutes
Servings: 2
Ingredients:

- 1 tablespoon extra-virgin olive oil
- 1 teaspoon cumin
- ½ finely diced red onion
- 1 minced garlic clove
- 1 teaspoon harissa spices
- 1 cup arugula
- 1 juiced lemon
- 6-ounce lean ground lamb
- 1 tablespoon parsley
- ½ cup low-fat plain yogurt

Directions:

1. Preheat the broiler on medium to high heat. Mix the ground lamb, red onion, parsley, Harissa spices, and olive oil until

combined.

2. Shape 1-inch thick patties using wet hands. Add the patties to a baking tray and place under the broiler for 7-8 minutes on each side. Mix the yogurt, lemon juice, and cumin and serve over the lamb burgers with arugula's side salad.

Nutrition: Calories 306 Fat 20g Carbs 10g Phosphorus 269mg Potassium 492mg Sodium 86mg Protein 23g

115. Pork Loins with Leeks

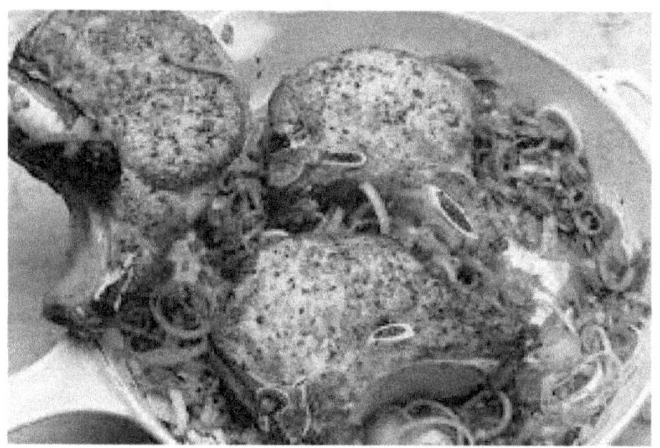

Preparation Time: 10 minutes
Cooking Time: 35 minutes
Servings: 2
Ingredients:

- 1 sliced leek
- 1 tablespoon mustard seeds
- 6-ounce pork tenderloin
- 1 tablespoon cumin seeds
- 1 tablespoon dry mustard
- 1 tablespoon extra-virgin oil

Directions:

1. Preheat the broiler to medium-high heat. In a dry skillet, heat mustard and cumin seeds until they start to pop (3-5 minutes). Grind seeds using a pestle and mortar or blender and then mix in the dry mustard.
2. Massage the pork on all sides using the mustard blend and add to a baking tray to broil for 25-30 minutes or until cooked through. Turn once halfway through.
3. Remove and place to one side, then heat-up the oil in a pan on medium heat and add the leeks for 5-6 minutes or until soft. Serve the pork tenderloin on a bed of leeks and enjoy it!

Nutrition: Calories 139 Fat 5g Carbs 2g Phosphorus 278mg Potassium 45mg Sodium 47mg Protein 18g

116. Chinese Beef Wraps

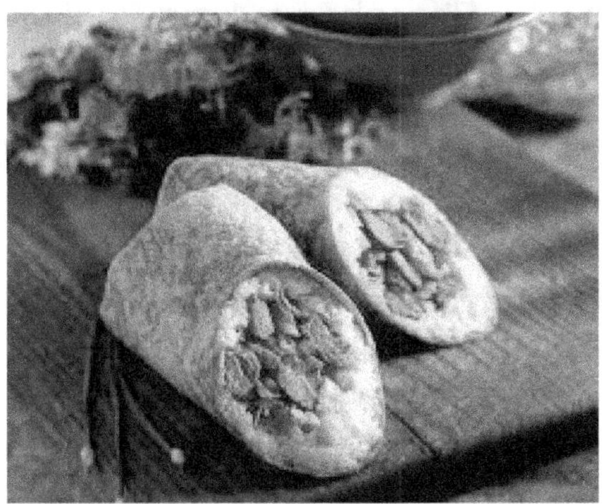

Preparation Time: 10 minutes
Cooking Time: 30 minutes
Servings: 2
Ingredients:

- 2 iceberg lettuce leaves
- ½ diced cucumber

- 1 teaspoon canola oil
- 5-ounce lean ground beef
- 1 teaspoon ground ginger
- 1 tablespoon chili flakes
- 1 minced garlic clove
- 1 tablespoon rice wine vinegar

Directions:

1. Mix the ground meat with the garlic, rice wine vinegar, chili flakes, and ginger in a bowl. Heat-up oil in a skillet over medium heat.
2. Put the beef in the pan and cook for 20-25 minutes or until cooked through. Serve beef mixture with diced cucumber in each lettuce wrap and fold.

Nutrition: Calories 156 Fat 2g Carbs 4 g Phosphorus 1 mg Sodium 54mg Protein 14g Potassium 0mg

117. Spicy Lamb Curry

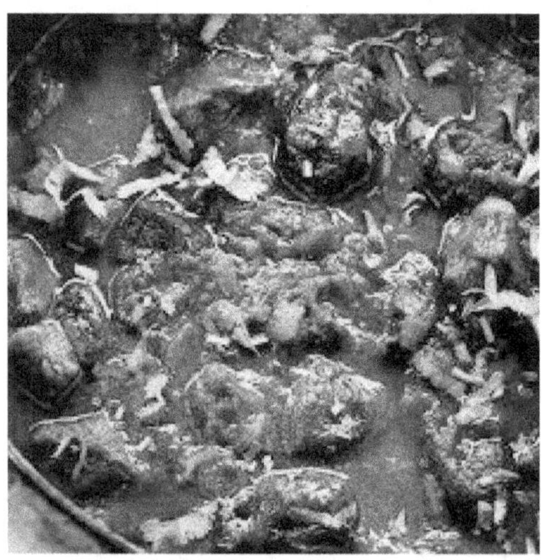

Preparation Time: 15 minutes
Cooking Time: 2 hours 15 minutes

Servings: 6-8
Ingredients:

- 4 teaspoons ground coriander
- 4 teaspoons ground coriander
- 4 teaspoons ground cumin
- ¾ teaspoon ground ginger
- 2 teaspoons ground cinnamon
- ½ teaspoon ground cloves
- ½ teaspoon ground cardamom
- 2 tablespoons sweet paprika
- ½ tablespoon cayenne pepper
- 2 teaspoons chili powder
- 2 teaspoons salt
- 1 tablespoon coconut oil
- 2 pounds boneless lamb, trimmed and cubed into 1-inch size
- Salt
- ground black pepper
- 2 cups onions, chopped
- 1¼ cups water
- 1 cup of coconut almond milk

Directions:

1. For spice mixture in a bowl, mix all spices. Keep aside. Season the lamb with salt and black pepper.
2. Warm oil on medium-high heat in a large Dutch oven. Add lamb and stir fry for around 5 minutes. Add onion and cook approximately 4-5 minutes.
3. Stir in the spice mixture and cook approximately 1 minute. Add water and coconut almond milk and provide some boil on high heat.

4. Adjust the heat to low and simmer, covered for approximately 1-120 minutes or until the lamb's desired doneness. Uncover and simmer for about 3-4 minutes. Serve hot.

Nutrition: Calories: 466 Fat: 10g Carbohydrates: 23g Protein: 36g Potassium 599 mg Sodium 203 mg Phosphorus 0mg

118. Roast Beef

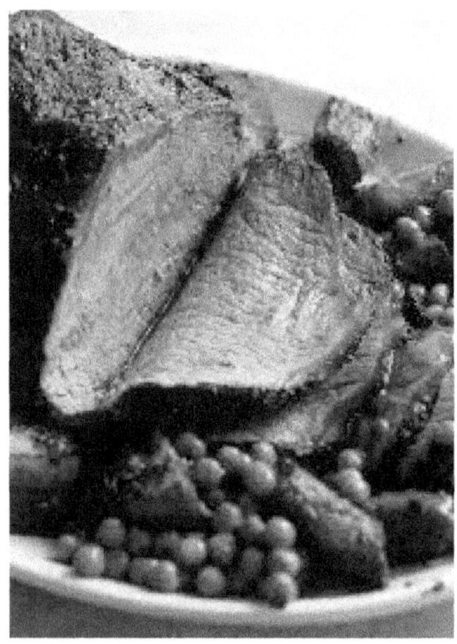

Preparation Time: 25 minutes
Cooking Time: 55 minutes
Servings: 3
Ingredients:

- Quality rump or sirloin tip roast
- Pepper & herbs

Directions:

1. Place in a roasting pan on a shallow rack. Season with pepper and herbs. Insert meat thermometer in the center or thickest part of the roast.
2. Roast to the desired degree of doneness. After removing from over for about 15 minutes, let it chill. In the end, the roast should be moister than well done.

Nutrition: Calories 158 Protein 24 g Fat 6 g Carbs 0 g Phosphorus 206 mg Potassium 328 mg Sodium 55 mg
492.

119. Grilled Skirt Steak

Preparation Time: 15 minutes
Cooking Time: 8-9 minutes
Servings: 4
Ingredients:

- 2 teaspoons fresh ginger herb, grated finely
- 2 teaspoons fresh lime zest, grated finely
- 1/4 cup coconut sugar
- 2 teaspoons fish sauce
- 2 tablespoons fresh lime juice
- 1/2 cup coconut almond milk
- 1-pound beef skirt steak, trimmed and cut into 4-inch slices lengthwise
- Salt, to taste

Directions:

1. In a sizable sealable bag, mix together all ingredients except steak and salt.
2. Add steak and coat with marinade generously.
3. Seal the bag and refrigerate to marinate for about 4-12 hours.

4. Preheat the grill to high heat. Grease the grill grate.
5. Remove steak from refrigerator and discard the marinade.
6. With a paper towel, dry the steak and sprinkle with salt evenly.
7. Cook the steak for approximately 31/2 minutes.
8. Flip the medial side and cook for around 21/2-5 minutes or till desired doneness.
9. Remove from grill pan and keep side for approximately 5 minutes before slicing.
10. With a clear, crisp knife cut into desired slices and serve.

Nutrition: Calories: 465, Fat: 10g, Carbohydrates: 22g, Fiber: 0g, Protein: 37g

120. Lamb with Zucchini & Couscous

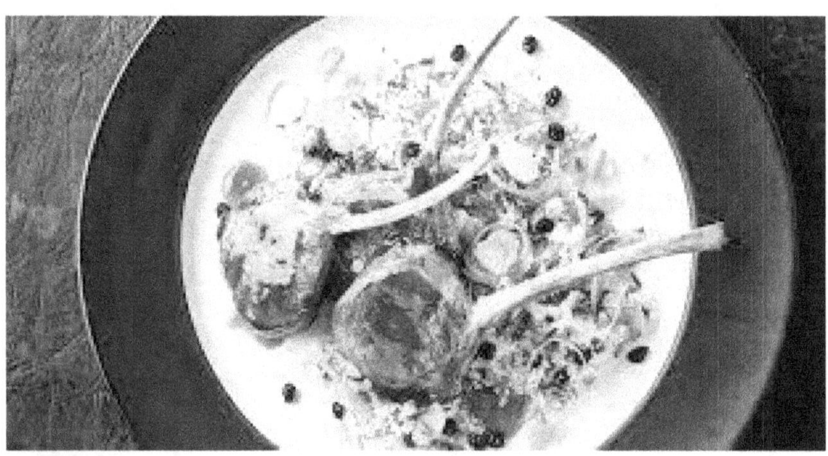

Preparation Time: 15 minutes
Cooking Time: 8 minutes
Servings: 2
Ingredients:

- ¾ cup couscous

- ¾ cup boiling water
- 1/4 cup fresh cilantro, chopped
- 1 tbsp. olive oil
- 5-ounces lamb leg steak, cubed into ¾-inch size
- 1 medium zucchini, sliced thinly
- 1 medium red onion, cut into wedges
- 1 teaspoon ground cumin
- 1 teaspoon ground coriander
- 1/4 teaspoon red pepper flakes, crushed
- Salt, to taste
- 1/4 cup plain Greek yogurt
- 1 garlic herb, minced

Directions:

1. In a bowl, add couscous and boiling water and stir to combine,
2. Cover whilst aside approximately 5 minutes.
3. Add cilantro and with a fork, fluff completely.
4. Meanwhile in a substantial skillet, heat oil on high heat.
5. Add lamb and stir fry for about 2-3 minutes.
6. Add zucchini and onion and stir fry for about 2 minutes.
7. Stir in spices and stir fry for about 1 minute
8. Add couscous and stir fry approximately 2 minutes.
9. In a bowl, mix together yogurt and garlic.
10. Divide lamb mixture in serving plates evenly.
11. Serve using the topping of yogurt.

Nutrition: Calories: 392, Fat: 5g, Carbohydrates: 2g, Fiber: 12g, Protein: 35g

121. Lemon Butter Salmon

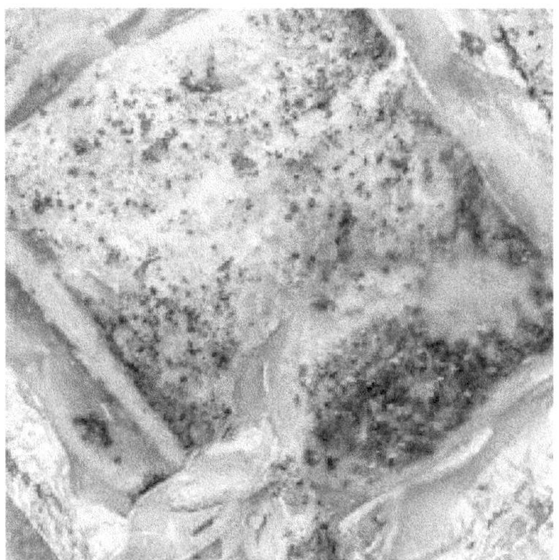

Preparation Time: 15 minutes
Cooking Time: 15 minutes
Servings: 6
Ingredients:

- 1 tbsp. butter
- 2 tbsps. olive oil
- 1 tbsp. Dijon mustard
- 1 tbsp. lemon juice
- 2 cloves garlic, crushed
- 1 tsp. dried dill
- 1 tsp. dried basil leaves
- 1 tbsp. capers
- 24 oz. salmon filet

Directions:

1. Put all the ingredients except the salmon in a saucepan over medium heat.
2. Bring to a boil and then simmer for 5 minutes.
3. Preheat your grill.
4. Create a packet using foil.
5. Place the sauce and salmon inside.
6. Seal the packet.
7. Grill for 12 minutes.

Nutrition: Calories: 294 Protein: 23 g Carbohydrates: 1 g Fat: 22 g Cholesterol: 68 mg Sodium: 190 mg Potassium: 439 mg Phosphorus: 280 mg Calcium: 21 mg

122. Crab Cake

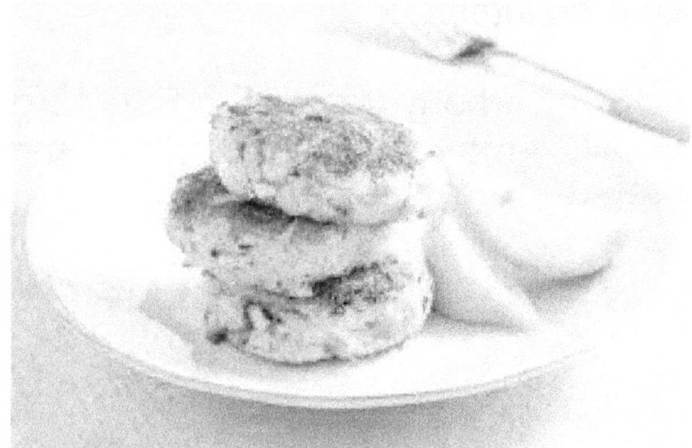

Preparation Time: 15 minutes
Cooking Time: 9 minutes
Servings: 6
Ingredients:

- ¼ cup onion, chopped
- ¼ cup bell pepper, chopped
- 1 egg, beaten
- 6 low-sodium crackers, crushed
- 1/4 cup low-fat mayonnaise

- 1 lb. crab meat
- 1 tbsp. dry mustard
- Pepper to taste
- 2 tbsps. lemon juice
- 1 tbsp. fresh parsley
- 1 tbsp. garlic powder
- 3 tbsps. olive oil

Directions:

1. Mix all the ingredients except the oil.
2. Form 6 patties from the mixture.
3. Pour the oil into a pan over medium heat.
4. Cook the crab cakes for 5 minutes.
5. Flip and cook for another 4 minutes.

Nutrition: Calories: 188 Protein: 13 g Carbohydrates: 5 g Fat: 13 g Cholesterol: 111 mg Sodium: 342 mg Potassium: 317 mg Phosphorus: 185 mg Calcium: 52 mg Fiber: 0.5 g

123. Baked Fish in Cream Sauce

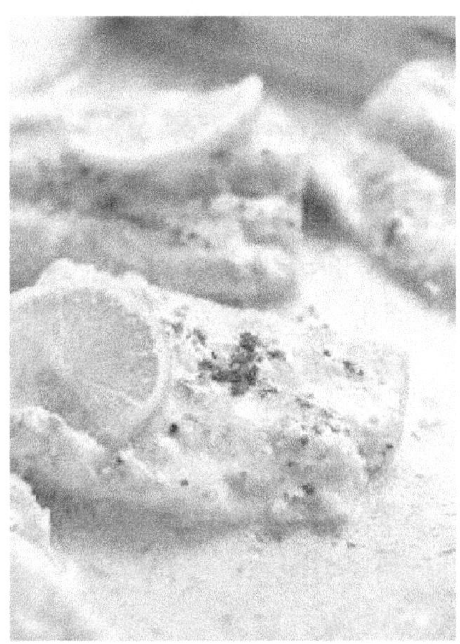

Preparation Time: 10 minutes
Cooking Time: 40 minutes
Servings: 4
Ingredients:

- 1 lb. haddock
- ½ cup all-purpose flour
- 2 tbsps. butter (unsalted)
- ¼ tsp. pepper
- 2 cups fat-free non-dairy creamer
- ¼ cup water

Directions:

1. Preheat your oven to 350° F.
2. Spray baking pan with oil.
3. Sprinkle with a little flour.
4. Arrange fish on the pan
5. Season with pepper.
6. Sprinkle remaining flour on the fish.

7. Spread creamer on both sides of the fish.
8. Bake for 40 minutes or until golden.
9. Spread cream sauce on top of the fish before serving.

Nutrition: Calories: 380 Protein: 23 g Carbohydrates: 46 g Fat: 11 g Cholesterol: 79 mg Sodium: 253 mg Potassium: 400 mg Phosphorus: 266 mg Calcium: 46 mg Fiber: 0.4 g

124. Shrimp & Broccoli

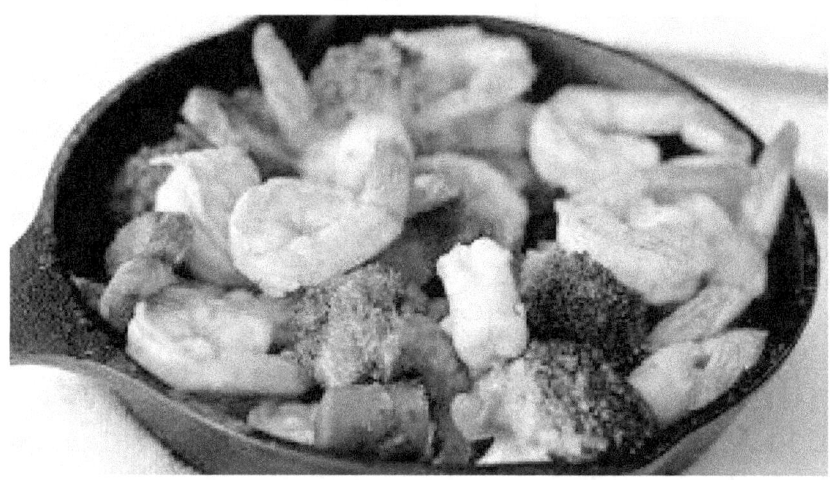

Preparation Time: 10 minutes
Cooking Time: 5 minutes
Servings: 4
Ingredients:

- 1 tbsp. olive oil
- 1 clove garlic, minced
- 1 lb. shrimp
- ¼ cup red bell pepper
- 1 cup broccoli florets, steamed
- 10 oz. cream cheese
- ½ tsp. garlic powder
- ¼ cup lemon juice

- ¾ tsp. ground peppercorns
- ¼ cup half and half creamer

Directions:

1. In a pan over medium heat, pour the oil and cook garlic for 30 seconds.
2. Add shrimp and cook for 2 minutes.
3. Add the rest of the ingredients.
4. Mix well.
5. Cook for 2 minutes.

Nutrition: Calories: 468 Protein: 27 g Carbohydrates: 28 g Fat: 28 g Cholesterol: 213 mg Sodium: 374 mg Potassium: 469 mg Phosphorus: 335 mg Calcium: 157 mg Fiber: 2.6 g

125. Shrimp in Garlic Sauce

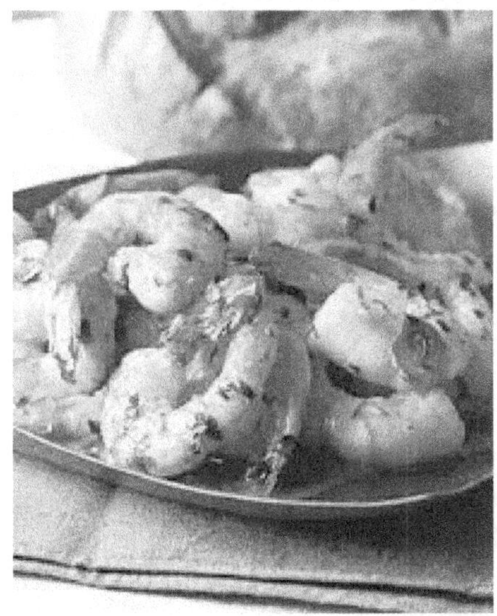

Preparation Time: 10 minutes
Cooking Time: 6 minutes
Servings: 4
Ingredients:

- 3 tbsps. butter (unsalted)
- ¼ cup onion, minced
- 3 cloves garlic, minced
- 1 lb. shrimp, shelled and deveined
- ½ cup half and half creamer
- ¼ cup white wine
- 2 tbsps. fresh basil
- Black pepper to taste

Directions:

1. Add butter to a pan over medium-low heat.
2. Let it melt.
3. Add the onion and garlic.
4. Cook for 1 minute.
5. Add the shrimp and cook for 2 minutes.
6. Transfer shrimp on a serving platter and set aside.
7. Add the rest of the ingredients.
8. Simmer for 3 minutes.
9. Pour sauce over the shrimp and serve.

Nutrition: Calories: 483 Protein: 32 g Carbohydrates: 46 g Fat: 19 g Cholesterol: 230 mg Sodium: 213 mg Potassium: 514 mg Phosphorus: 398 mg Calcium: 133 mg Fiber: 2.0 g

126. Fish Taco

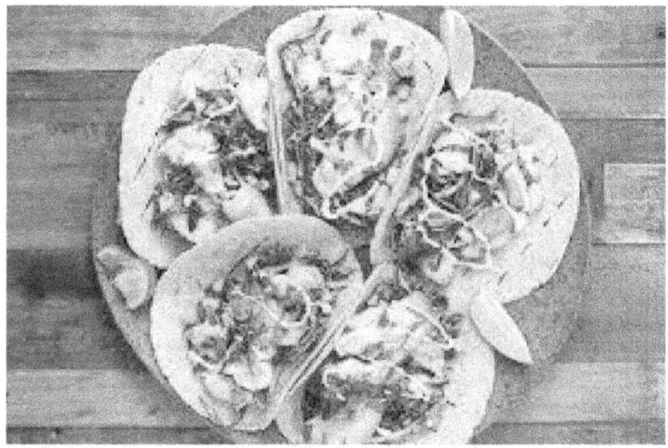

Preparation Time: 40 minutes
Cooking Time: 10 minutes
Servings: 6
Ingredients:

- 1 tbsp. lime juice
- 1 tbsp. olive oil
- 1 clove garlic, minced
- 1 lb. cod fillets
- ½ tsp. ground cumin
- ¼ tsp. black pepper
- ½ tsp. chili powder
- ¼ cup sour cream
- ½ cup mayonnaise
- 2 tbsps. nondairy milk
- 1 cup cabbage, shredded
- ½ cup onion, chopped
- ½ bunch cilantro, chopped
- 12 corn tortillas

Directions:

1. Drizzle lemon juice over the fish fillet.

2. Coat with olive oil and season with garlic, cumin, pepper and chili powder.
3. Let it sit for 30 minutes.
4. Broil fish for 10 minutes, flipping halfway through.
5. Flake the fish using a fork.
6. In a bowl, mix sour cream, milk and mayo.
7. Assemble tacos by filling each tortilla with mayo mixture, cabbage, onion, cilantro and fish flakes.

Nutrition: Calories: 363 Protein: 18 g Carbohydrates: 30 g Fat: 19 g Cholesterol: 40 mg Sodium: 194 mg Potassium: 507 mg Phosphorus: 327 mg Calcium: 138 mg Fiber: 4.3 g

127. Baked Trout

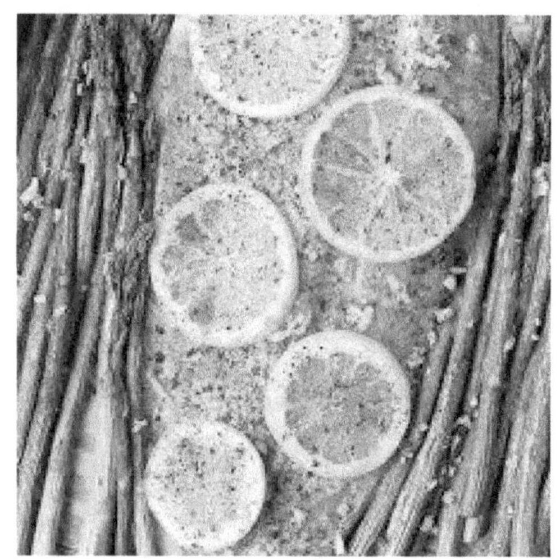

Preparation Time: 5 minutes
Cooking Time: 10 minutes
Servings: 8
Ingredients:

- 2 lb. trout fillet
- 1 tbsp. oil
- 1 tsp. salt-free lemon pepper

- ½ tsp. paprika

Directions:

1. Preheat your oven to 350° F.
2. Coat fillet with oil.
3. Place fish on a baking pan.
4. Season with lemon pepper and paprika.
5. Bake for 10 minutes.

Nutrition: Calories: 161 Protein: 21 g Carbohydrates: 0 g Fat: 8 g Cholesterol: 58 mg Sodium: 109 mg Potassium: 385 mg Phosphorus: 227 mg Calcium: 75 mg Fiber: 0.1 g

128. Fish With Mushrooms

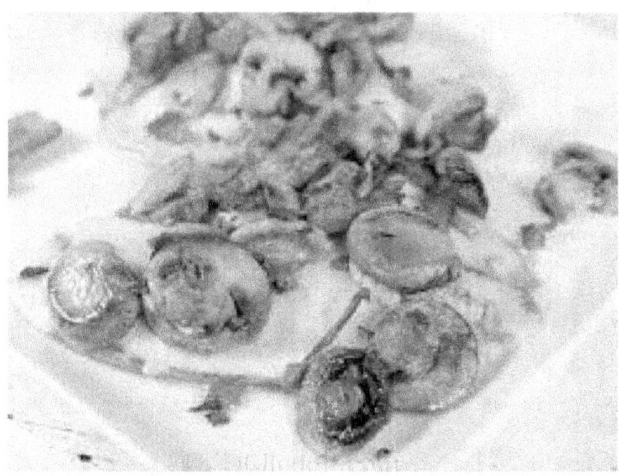

Preparation Time: 5 minutes
Cooking Time: 16 minutes
Servings: 4
Ingredients:

- 1 lb. cod fillet
- 2 tbsps. butter
- ¼ cup white onion, chopped
- 1 cup fresh mushrooms

- 1 tsp. dried thyme

Directions:

1. Put the fish in a baking pan.
2. Preheat your oven to 450° F.
3. In a pan over medium heat, melt the butter and cook onion and mushroom for 1 minute.
4. Spread mushroom mixture on top of the fish.
5. Season with thyme.
6. Bake in the oven for 15 minutes.

Nutrition: Calories: 155 Protein: 21 g Carbohydrates: 2 g Fat: 7 g Cholesterol: 49 mg Sodium: 110 mg Potassium: 561 mg Phosphorus: 225 mg Calcium: 30 mg

129. Saucy Dill Fish

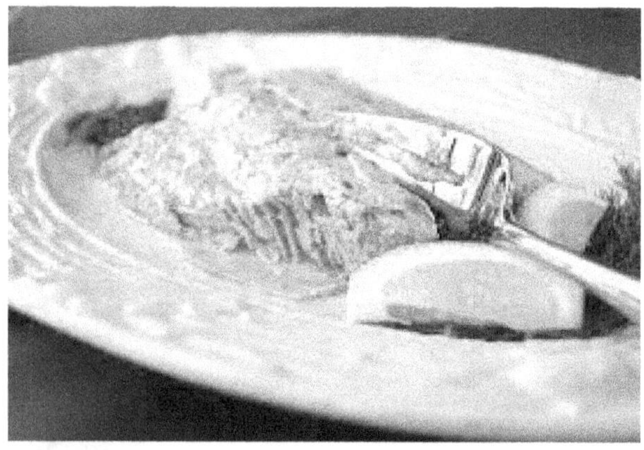

Preparation Time: 10 minutes
Cooking Time: 15 minutes
Servings: 4
Ingredients:

- 4 (4 oz.) salmon fillets

Dill Sauce:

- 1 cup whipped cream cheese
- 4 minced garlic cloves
- ½ small onion, diced
- 3 tbsps. fresh or dried dill (as desired)
- ½ tsp. ground pepper
- 1 tsp. Mrs. Dash (optional)
- 2 drops of hot sauce (optional)

Directions:

1. Place the salmon fillets in a moderately shallow baking stray.
2. Whisk the cream cheese and all the dill-sauce ingredients in a bowl.
3. Spread the dill-sauce over the fillets liberally.
4. Cover the fillet pan with a foil sheet and bake for 15 minutes at 350° F.
5. Serve warm.

Nutrition: Calories: 432 Total Fat: 26.7 g Saturated Fat: 12.9 g Cholesterol: 142 mg Sodium: 280 mg Carbohydrates: 5 g Phosphorus: 265 mg Potassium: 590 mg

130. Lemon Pepper Trout

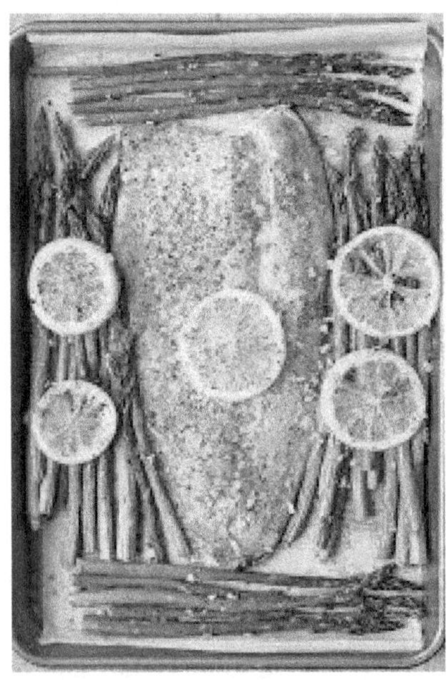

Preparation Time: 10 minutes
Cooking Time: 15 minutes
Servings: 2
Ingredients:

- 1 lb. trout fillets
- 1 lb. asparagus
- 3 tbsps. olive oil
- 5 garlic cloves, minced
- ½ tsp. black pepper
- ½ lemon, sliced

Directions:

1. Prepare and preheat the gas oven at 350° F.
2. Rub the washed and dried fillets with oil then place them in a baking tray.
3. Top the fish with lemon slices, black pepper, and garlic cloves.
4. Spread the asparagus around the fish.

5. Bake the fish for 15 minutes approximately in the preheated oven.
6. Serve warm.

Nutrition: Calories: 336 Total Fat: 20.3 g Saturated Fat: 3.2 g Cholesterol: 84 mg Sodium: 370 mg Carbohydrates: 6.5 g Phosphorus: 107 mg Potassium: 383 mg

131. Salmon Stuffed Pasta

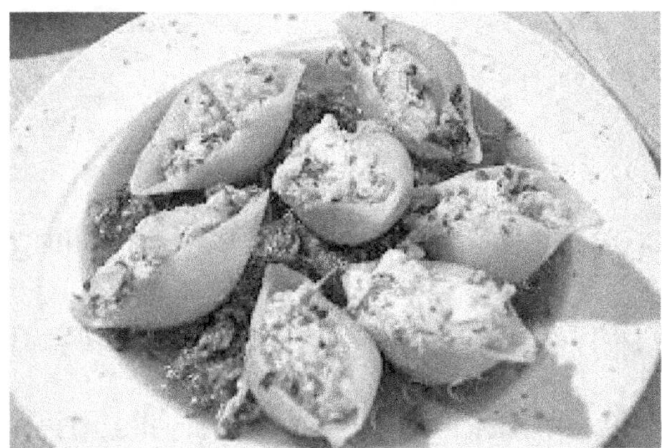

Preparation Time: 10 minutes
Cooking Time: 35 minutes
Servings: 24
Ingredients:

- 24 jumbo pasta shells, boiled
- 1 cup coffee creamer

Filling:

- 2 eggs, beaten
- 2 cups creamed cottage cheese
- ¼ cup chopped onion
- 1 red bell pepper, diced
- 2 tsps. dried parsley

* ½ tsp. lemon peel
* 1 can salmon, drained

Dill Sauce:

* 1 ½ tsp. butter
* 1 ½ tsp. flour
* 1/8 tsp. pepper
* 1 tbsp. lemon juice
* 1 ½ cup coffee creamer
* 2 tsps. dried dill weed

Directions:

1. Beat the egg with the cream cheese and all the other filling ingredients in a bowl.
2. Divide the filling in the pasta shells and place the shells in a 9x13 baking dish.
3. Pour the coffee creamer around the stuffed shells then cover with a foil.
4. Bake the shells for 30 minutes at 350° F.
5. Meanwhile, whisk all the ingredients for dill sauce in a saucepan.
6. Stir for 5 minutes until it thickens.
7. Pour this sauce over the baked pasta shells.
8. Serve warm.

Nutrition: Calories: 268 Total Fat: 4.8 g Saturated Fat: 2 g Cholesterol: 27 mg Sodium: 86 mg Total Carbohydrates: 42.6 g Phosphorus: 314 mg Potassium: 181 mg

132. Herbed Vegetable Trout

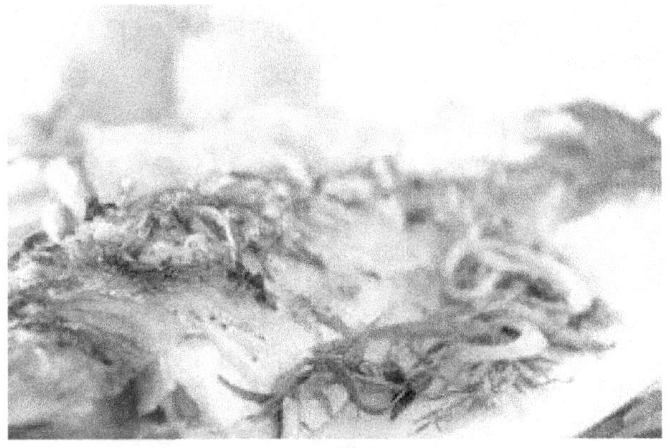

Preparation Time: 10 minutes
Cooking Time: 15 minutes
Servings: 4
Ingredients:

- 14 oz. trout fillets
- ½ tsp. herb seasoning blend
- 1 lemon, sliced
- 2 green onions, sliced
- 1 stalk celery, chopped
- 1 medium carrot, julienne

Directions:

1. Prepare and preheat a charcoal grill over moderate heat.
2. Place the trout fillets over a large piece of foil and drizzle herb seasoning on top.
3. Spread the lemon slices, carrots, celery, and green onions over the fish.
4. Cover the fish with foil and pack it.
5. Place the packed fish in the grill and cook for 15 minutes.
6. Once done, remove the foil from the fish.
7. Serve.

Nutrition: Calories: 202 Total Fat: 8.5 g Saturated Fat: 1.5 g Cholesterol: 73 mg Sodium: 82 mg Carbohydrates: 3.5 g Phosphorus: 287 mg Potassium: 560 mg

133. Citrus Glazed Salmon

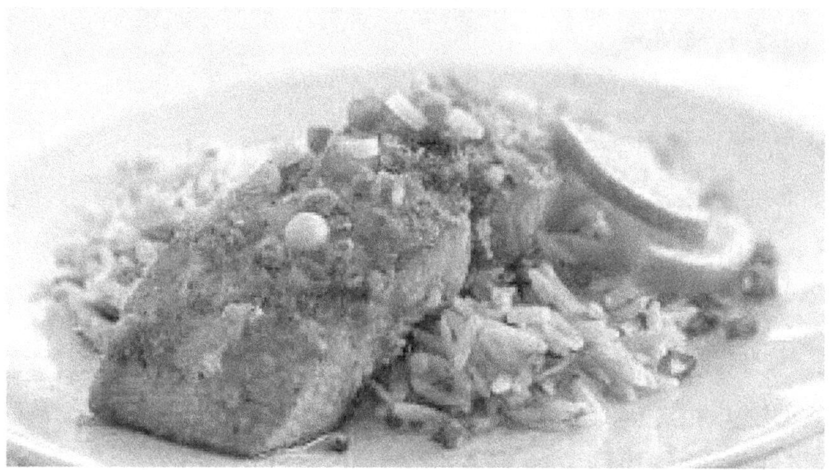

Preparation Time: 10 minutes
Cooking Time: 17 minutes
Servings: 2
Ingredients:

- 2 garlic cloves, crushed
- 1 ½ tbsps. lemon juice
- 2 tbsps. olive oil
- 1 tbsp. butter
- 1 tbsp. Dijon mustard
- 2 dashes of cayenne pepper
- 1 tsp. dried basil leaves
- 1 tsp. dried dill
- 24 oz. salmon filet

Directions:

1. Place a 1-quart saucepan over moderate heat and add the oil, butter, garlic, lemon juice, mustard, cayenne pepper, dill, and basil to the pan.
2. Stir this mixture for 5 minutes after it has boiled.
3. Prepare and preheat a charcoal grill over moderate heat.
4. Place the fish on a foil sheet and fold the edges to make a foil tray.
5. Pour the prepared sauce over the fish.
6. Place the fish in the foil in the preheated grill and cook for 12 minutes.
7. Slice and serve.

Nutrition: Calories: 401 Total Fat: 20.5 g Saturated Fat: 5.3 g Cholesterol: 144 mg Sodium: 256 mg Carbohydrates: 0.5 g Phosphorus: 214 mg Potassium: 446 mg

134. Broiled Salmon Fillets

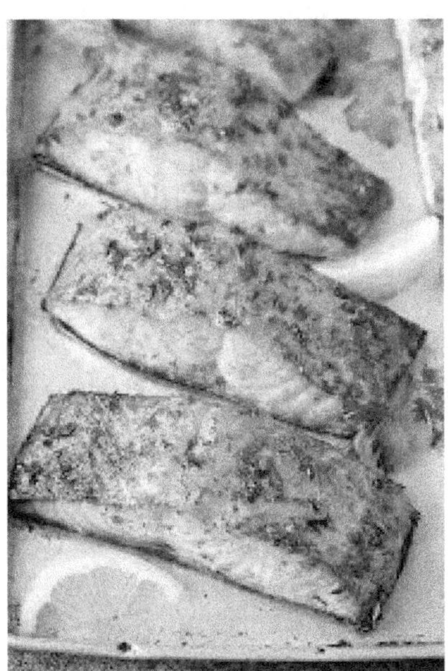

Preparation Time: 10 minutes
Cooking Time: 15 minutes

Servings: 4
Ingredients:

- 1 tbsp. ginger root, grated
- 1 clove garlic, minced
- ¼ cup maple syrup
- 1 tbsp. hot pepper sauce
- 4 salmon fillets, skinless

Directions:

1. Grease a pan with cooking spray and place it over moderate heat.
2. Add the ginger and garlic and sauté for 3 minutes then transfer to a bowl.
3. Add the hot pepper sauce and maple syrup to the ginger-garlic.
4. Mix well and keep this mixture aside.
5. Place the salmon fillet in a suitable baking tray, greased with cooking oil.
6. Brush the maple sauce over the fillets liberally
7. Broil them for 10 minutes in the oven at broiler settings.
8. Serve warm.

Nutrition: Calories: 289 Total Fat: 11.1 g Saturated Fat: 1.6 g Cholesterol: 78 mg Sodium: 80 mg Carbohydrates: 13.6 g Phosphorus: 230 mg Potassium: 331 mg

135. Broiled Shrimp

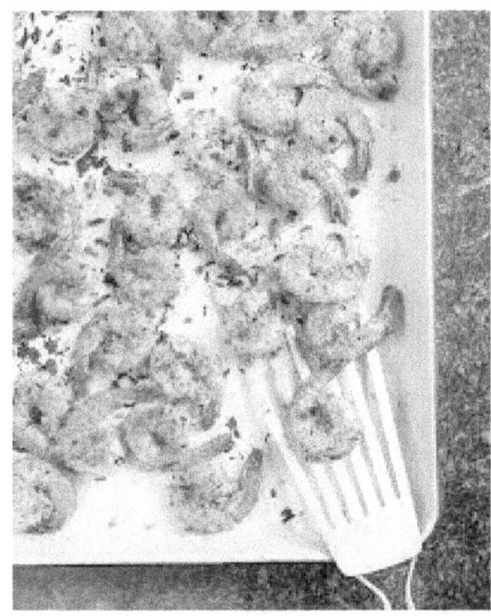

Preparation Time: 10 minutes
Cooking Time: 5 minutes
Servings: 2
Ingredients:

- 1 lb. shrimp in shell
- ½ cup unsalted butter, melted
- 2 tsps. lemon juice
- 2 tbsps. chopped onion
- 1 clove garlic, minced
- 1/8 tsp. pepper

Directions:

1. Toss the shrimp with butter, lemon juice, onion, garlic, and pepper in a bowl.
2. Spread the seasoned shrimp in a baking tray.
3. Broil for 5 minutes in an oven on a broiler setting.
4. Serve warm.

136. Grilled Lemony Cod

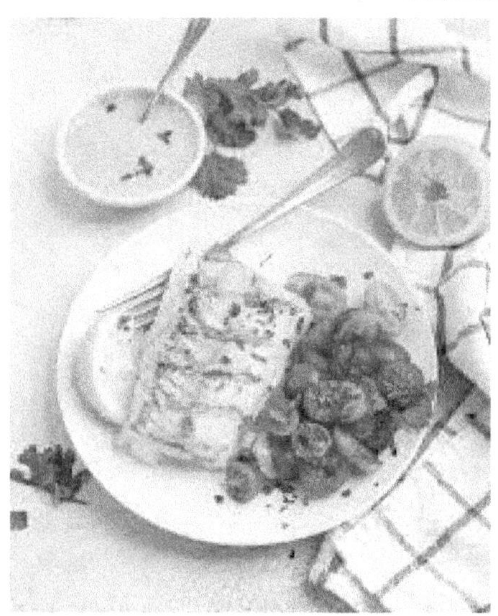

Preparation Time: 10 minutes
Cooking Time: 10 minutes
Servings: 4
Ingredients:

- 1 lb. cod fillets
- 1 tsp. salt-free lemon pepper seasoning
- ¼ cup lemon juice

Directions:

1. Rub the cod fillets with lemon pepper seasoning and lemon juice.
2. Grease a baking tray with cooking spray and place the salmon in the baking tray.

3. Bake the fish for 10 minutes at 350° F in a preheated oven.
4. Serve warm.

Nutrition: Calories: 155 Total Fat: 7.1 g Saturated Fat: 1.1 g Cholesterol: 50 mg Sodium: 53 mg Carbohydrates: 0.7 g Calcium: 43 mg Phosphorus: 237 mg Potassium: 461 mg

137. Spiced Honey Salmon

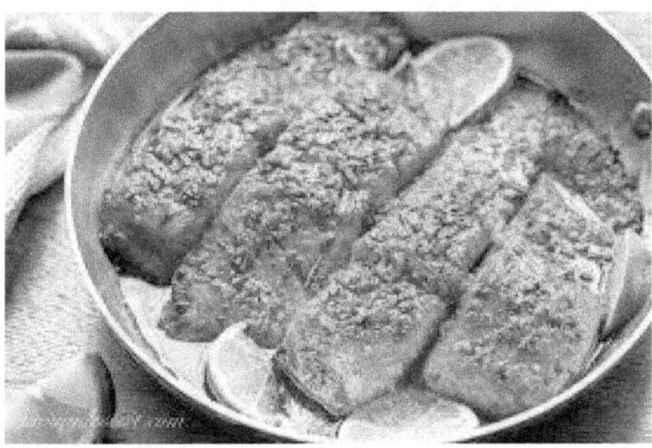

Preparation Time: 10 minutes
Cooking Time: 16 minutes
Servings: 2
Ingredients:

- 3 tbsps. honey
- ¾ tsp. lemon peel
- ½ tsp. black pepper
- ½ tsp. garlic powder
- 1 tsp. water
- 16 oz. salmon fillets
- 2 tbsps. olive oil
- Dill, chopped, to serve

Directions:

1. Whisk the lemon peel with honey, garlic powder, hot water, and ground pepper in a small bowl.
2. Rub this honey mixture over the salmon fillet liberally.
3. Set a suitable skillet over moderate heat and add olive oil to heat.
4. Set the spiced salmon fillets in the pan and sear them for 4 minutes per side.
5. Garnish with dill.
6. Serve warm.

Nutrition: Calories: 264 Total Fat: 14.1 g Saturated Fat: 2 g Cholesterol: 50 mg Sodium: 55 mgCarbohydrates: 14 g Calcium: 67 mg Phosphorus: 174 mg Potassium: 507 mg

138. Oregon Tuna Patties

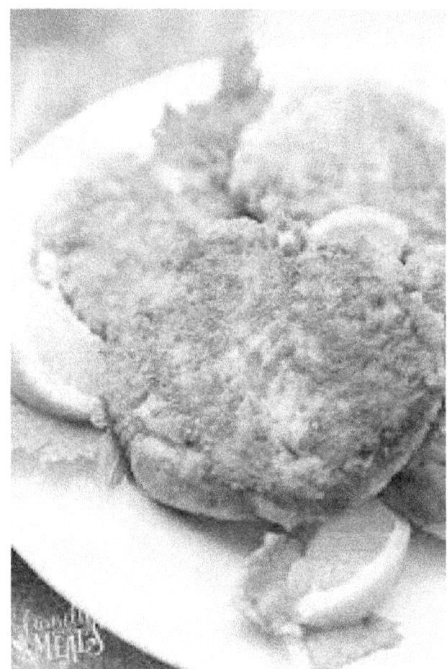

Preparation Time: 10 minutes
Cooking Time: 15 minutes
Servings: 4
Ingredients:

- 1 (14.75 ounce) can of tuna
- 2 tbsps. butter
- 1 medium onion, chopped
- 2/3 cup graham cracker crumbs
- 2 egg whites, beaten
- ¼ cup chopped fresh parsley
- 1 tsp. dry mustard
- 3 tbsps. olive oil

Directions:

1. Drain the tuna, reserving 3/4 cup of the liquid. Flake the meat. Melt butter in a large skillet over medium-high heat. Add onion, and cook until tender.
2. In a medium bowl, combine the onions with the reserved tuna liquid, 1/3 of the graham cracker crumbs, egg whites, parsley, mustard and tuna.
3. Heat olive in a large skillet over medium heat. Cook patties until browned, then carefully turn and brown on the other side.

Nutrition: Calories: 204 Total Fat: 15.4 g Saturated Fat: 4.4 g
Cholesterol: 74 mg Sodium: 111 mg
Total Carbohydrates: 6.5 g Potassium: 164 mg Phosphorus: 106 mg

139. Fish Chowder

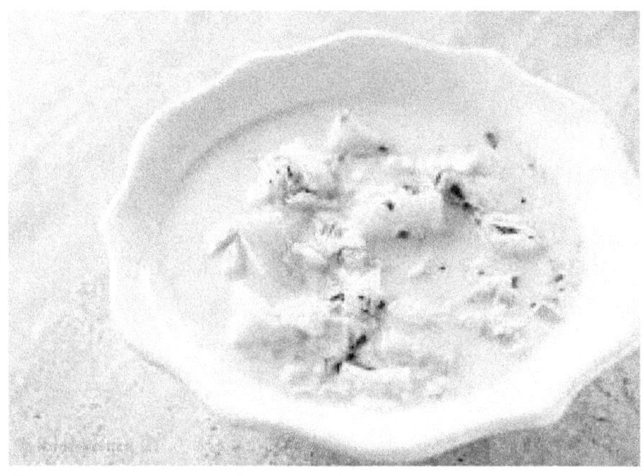

Preparation Time: 20 minutes
Cooking Time: 40 minutes
Servings: 4
Ingredients:

- 2 tbsps. butter
- 2 cups chopped onion
- 4 fresh mushrooms, sliced
- 1 stalk celery, chopped
- 4 cups chicken stock
- 2 lbs. cod, diced into 1/2-inch cubes
- ½ cup all-purpose flour
- 1/8 tsp. salt-free seasoning, or to taste \
- Ground black pepper to taste
- 2 (12 fluid ounce) cans soy milk

Directions:

1. In a large stockpot, melt 2 tbsps. butter over medium heat. Sauté onions, mushrooms, and celery in butter until tender.
2. Add chicken stock simmer for 10 minutes.
3. Add cod, and simmer another 10 minutes.

4. Mix flour until smooth; stir into soup and simmer for 1 minute more. Season to taste with seasoning, and pepper. Remove from heat, and stir in soy milk.

Nutrition: Calories: 171 Total Fat: 4.2 g Saturated Fat: 2.1 g Cholesterol: 32 mg Sodium: 810 mg Total Carbohydrates: 19.3 g Potassium: 204 mg Phosphorus: 106 mg

140. Spiced Peaches

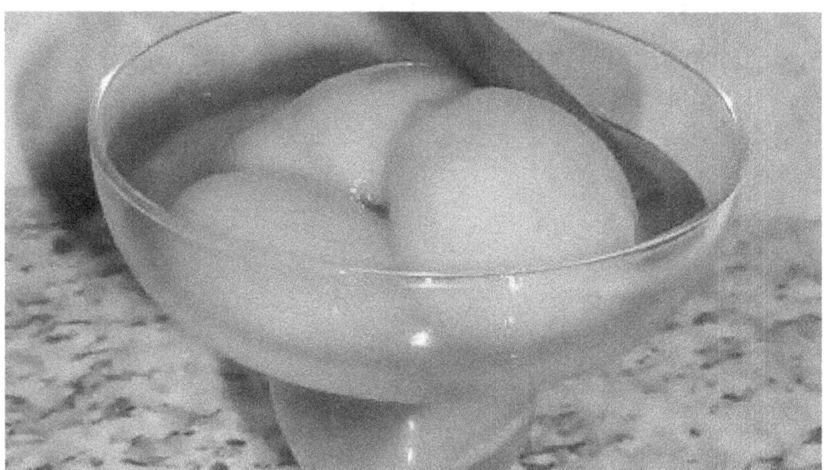

Preparation time: 5 minutes
Cooking time: 10 minutes
Servings: 2
Ingredients

- Canned peaches with juices – 1 cup
- Cornstarch – ½ tsp.
- Ground cloves – 1 tsp.
- Ground cinnamon – 1 tsp.
- Ground nutmeg – 1 tsp.
- Zest of ½ lemon
- Water – ½ cup

Direction:

1. Drain peaches.
2. Combine cinnamon, cornstarch, nutmeg, ground cloves, and lemon zest in a pan on the stove.

3. Heat on a medium heat and add peaches.
4. Bring to a boil, reduce the heat and simmer for 10 minutes.
5. Serve.

Nutrition Per Serving Calories: 70 Fat: 0g Carb: 14g Phosphorus: 23mg Potassium: 176mg Sodium: 3mg Protein: 1g

141. Pumpkin Cheesecake Bar

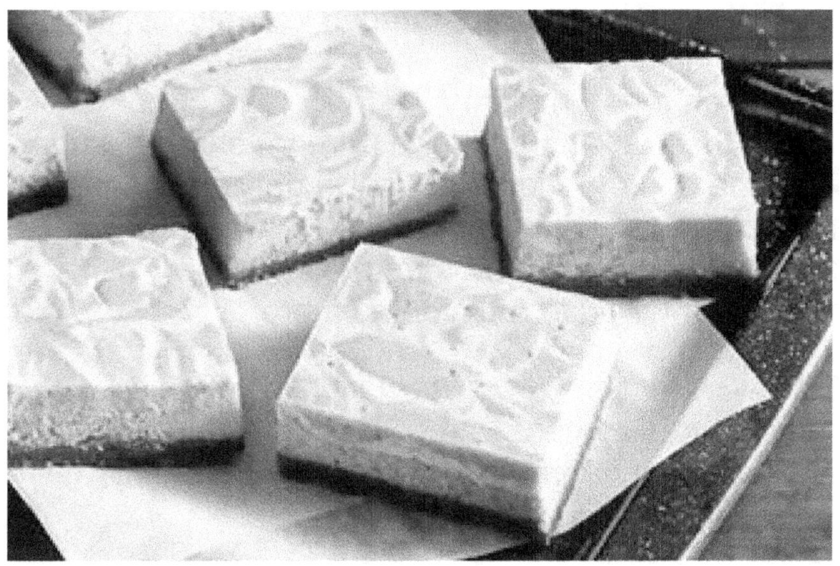

Preparation time: 10 minutes
Cooking time: 50 minutes
Servings: 4
Ingredients

- Unsalted butter – 2 ½ Tbsps.
- Cream cheese – 4 oz.
- All-purpose white flour – ½ cup
- Golden brown sugar – 3 Tbsps.
- Granulated sugar – ¼ cup
- Pureed pumpkin – ½ cup

- Egg whites - 2
- Ground cinnamon – 1 tsp.
- Ground nutmeg – 1 tsp.
- Vanilla extract – 1 tsp.

Direction:

1. Preheat the oven to 350F.
2. Mix flour and brown sugar in a bowl.
3. Mix in the butter to form 'breadcrumbs'.
4. Place ¾ of this mixture in a dish.
5. Bake in the oven for 15 minutes. Remove and cool.
6. Lightly whisk the egg and fold in the cream cheese, sugar, pumpkin, cinnamon, nutmeg and vanilla until smooth.
7. Pour this mixture over the oven-baked base and sprinkle with the rest of the breadcrumbs from earlier.
8. Bake in the oven for 30 to 35 minutes more.
9. Cool, slice and serve.

Nutrition Per Serving Calories: 248 Fat: 13g Carb: 33g Phosphorus: 67mg Potassium: 96mg Sodium: 146mg Protein: 4g

142. Blueberry Mini Muffins

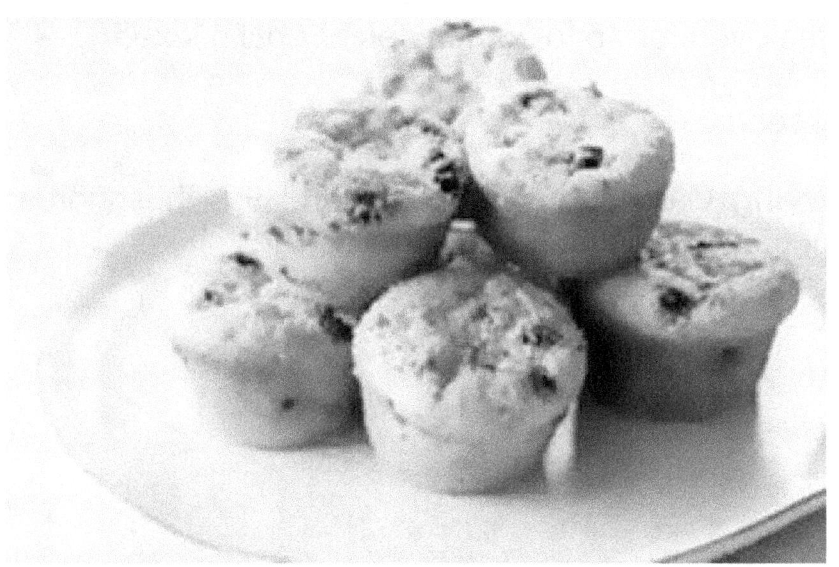

Preparation time: 10 minutes
Cooking time: 35 minutes
Servings: 4
Ingredients

- Egg whites – 3
- All-purpose white flour – ¼ cup
- Coconut flour – 1 Tbsp.
- Baking soda – 1 tsp.
- Nutmeg – 1 Tbsp. grated
- Vanilla extract – 1 tsp.
- Stevia – 1 tsp.
- Fresh blueberries – ¼ cup

Direction:

1. Preheat the oven to 325F.
2. Mix all the ingredients in a bowl.
3. Divide the batter into 4 and spoon into a lightly oiled muffin tin.

4. Bake in the oven for 15 to 20 minutes or until cooked through.
5. Cool and serve.

Nutrition Per Serving Calories: 62 Fat: 0g Carb: 9g Phosphorus: 103mg Potassium: 65mg Sodium: 62mg Protein: 4g

143. Vanilla Custard

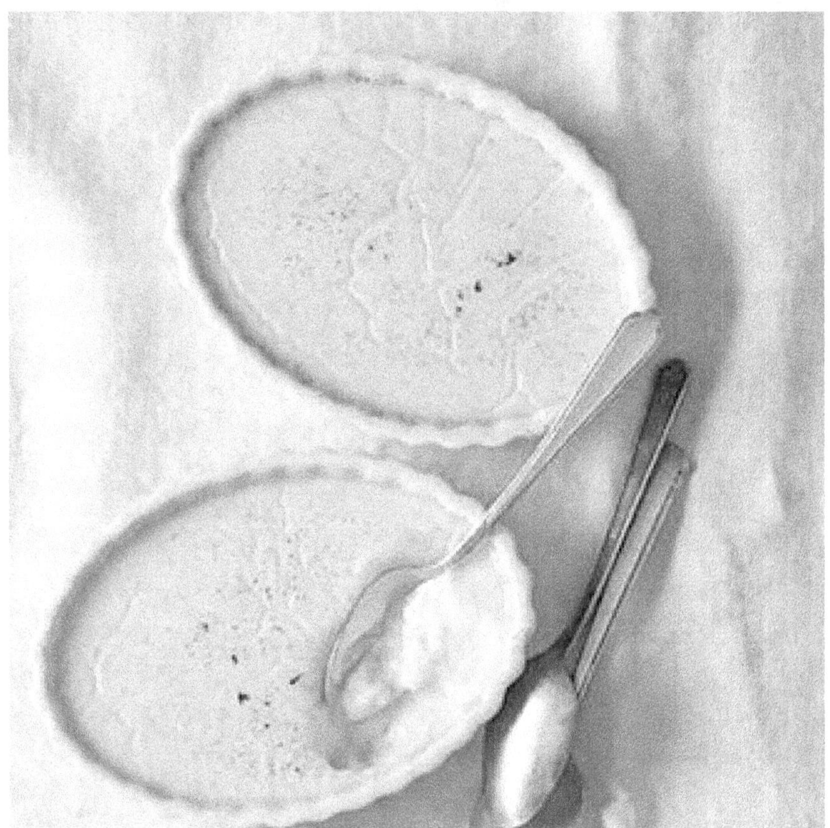

Preparation time: 7 minutes
Cooking time: 10 minutes
Servings: 10
Ingredients

- Egg – 1

- Vanilla – 1/8 tsp.
- Nutmeg – 1/8 tsp.
- Almond milk – ½ cup
- Stevia - 2 Tbsp.

Direction:

1. Scald the milk then let it cool slightly.
2. Break the egg into a bowl and beat it with the nutmeg.
3. Add the scalded milk, the vanilla, and the sweetener to taste. Mix well.
4. Place the bowl in a baking pan filled with ½ deep of water.
5. Bake for 30 minutes at 325F.
6. Serve.

Nutrition Per Serving Calories: 167.3 Fat: 9g Carb: 11g Phosphorus: 205mg Potassium: 249mg Sodium: 124mg Protein: 10g

144. Chocolate Chip Cookies

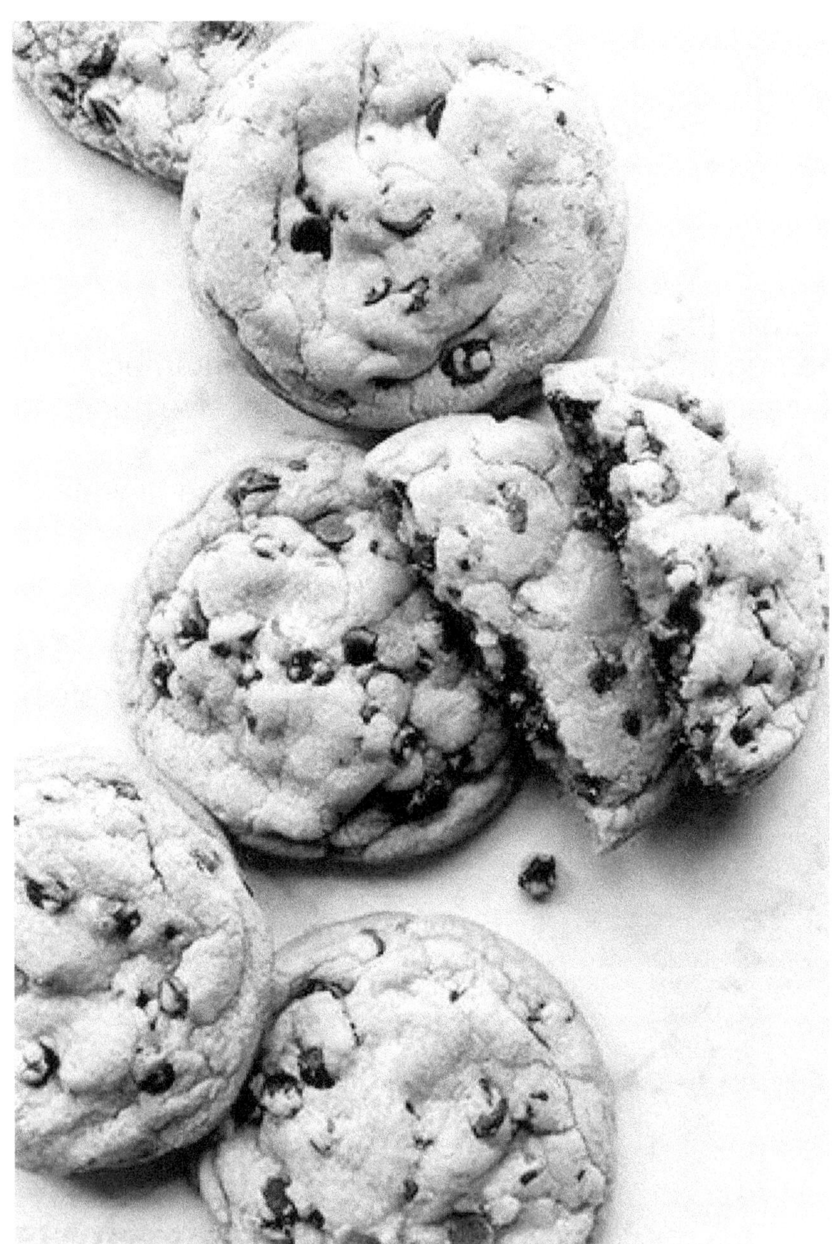

Preparation time: 7 minutes
Cooking time: 10 minutes
Servings: 10
Ingredients

- Semi-sweet chocolate chips – ½ cup
- Baking soda – ½ tsp.
- Vanilla – ½ tsp.
- Egg – 1
- Flour – 1 cup
- Margarine – ½ cup
- Stevia – 4 tsp.

Direction:

1. Sift the dry ingredients.
2. Cream the margarine, stevia, vanilla and egg with a whisk.
3. Add flour mixture and beat well.
4. Stir in the chocolate chips, then drop teaspoonfuls of the mixture over a greased baking sheet.
5. Bake the cookies for about 10 minutes at 375F.
6. Cool and serve.

Nutrition Per Serving Calories: 106.2 Fat: 7g Carb: 8.9g Phosphorus: 19mg Potassium: 28mg Sodium: 98mg Protein: 1.5g

145. Baked Peaches with Cream Cheese

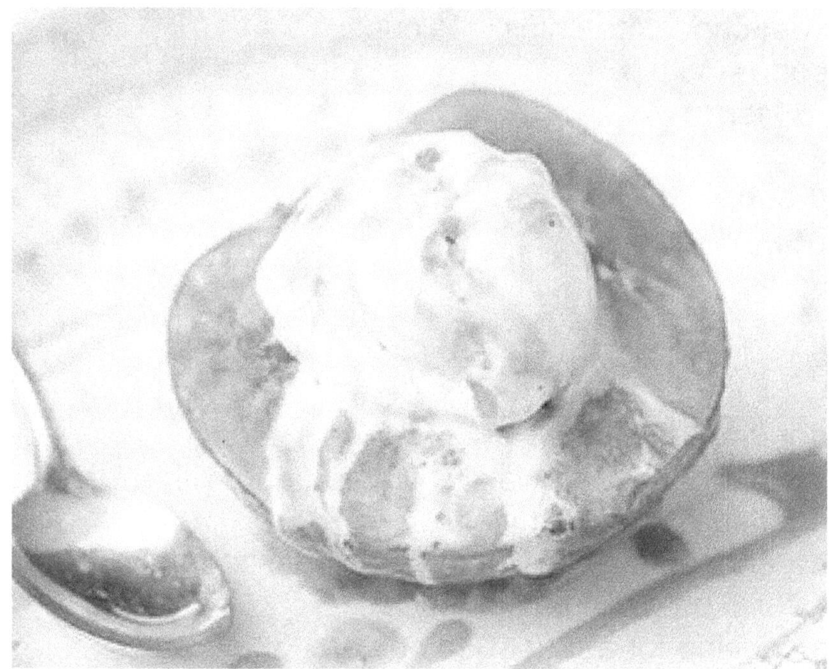

Preparation time: 10 minutes
Cooking time: 15 minutes
Servings: 4
Ingredients

- Plain cream cheese – 1 cup
- Crushed meringue cookies – ½ cup
- Ground cinnamon – ¼ tsp.
- Pinch ground nutmeg
- Canned peach halves – 8, in juice
- Honey – 2 Tbsp.

Direction:

1. Preheat the oven to 350F.
2. Line a baking sheet with parchment paper. Set aside.
3. In a small bowl, stir together the meringue cookies, cream cheese, cinnamon, and nutmeg.

4. Spoon the cream cheese mixture evenly into the cavities in the peach halves.
5. Place the peaches on the baking sheet and bake for 15 minutes or until the fruit is soft and the cheese is melted.
6. Remove the peaches from the baking sheet onto plates.
7. Drizzle with honey and serve.

Nutrition Per Serving Calories: 260 Fat: 20g Carb: 19g Phosphorus: 74mg Potassium: 198mg Sodium: 216mg Protein: 4g

146. Bread Pudding

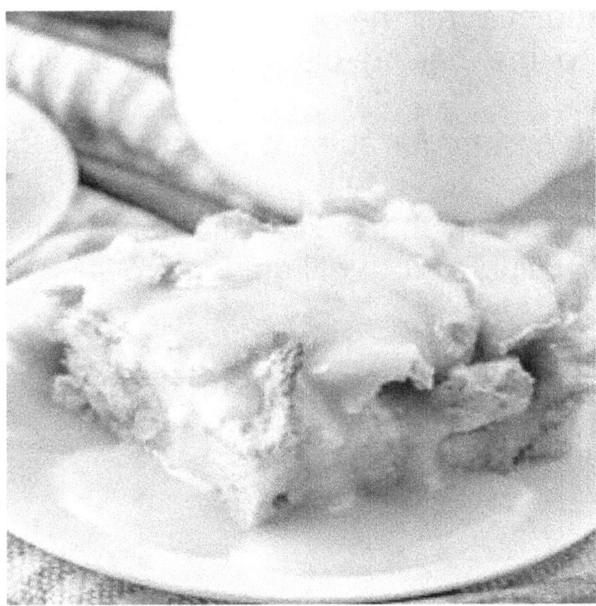

Preparation time: 15 minutes
Cooking time: 40 minutes
Servings: 6
Ingredients

- Unsalted butter, for greasing the baking dish
- Plain rice milk – 1 ½ cups
- Eggs – 2

- Egg whites – 2
- Honey – ¼ cup
- Pure vanilla extract – 1 tsp.
- Cubed white bread – 6 cups

Direction:

1. Lightly grease an 8-by-8-inch baking dish with butter. Set aside.
2. In a bowl, whisk together the eggs, egg whites, rice milk, honey, and vanilla.
3. Add the bread cubes and stir until the bread is coated.
4. Transfer the mixture to the baking dish and cover with plastic wrap.
5. Store the dish in the refrigerator for at least 3 hours.
6. Preheat the oven to 325F.
7. Remove the plastic wrap from the baking dish and bake the pudding for 35 to 40 minutes, or until golden brown.
8. Serve.

NutritionPer Serving Calories: 167 Fat: 3g Carb: 30g Phosphorus: 95mg Potassium: 93mg Sodium: 189mg Protein: 6g

147. Strawberry Ice Cream

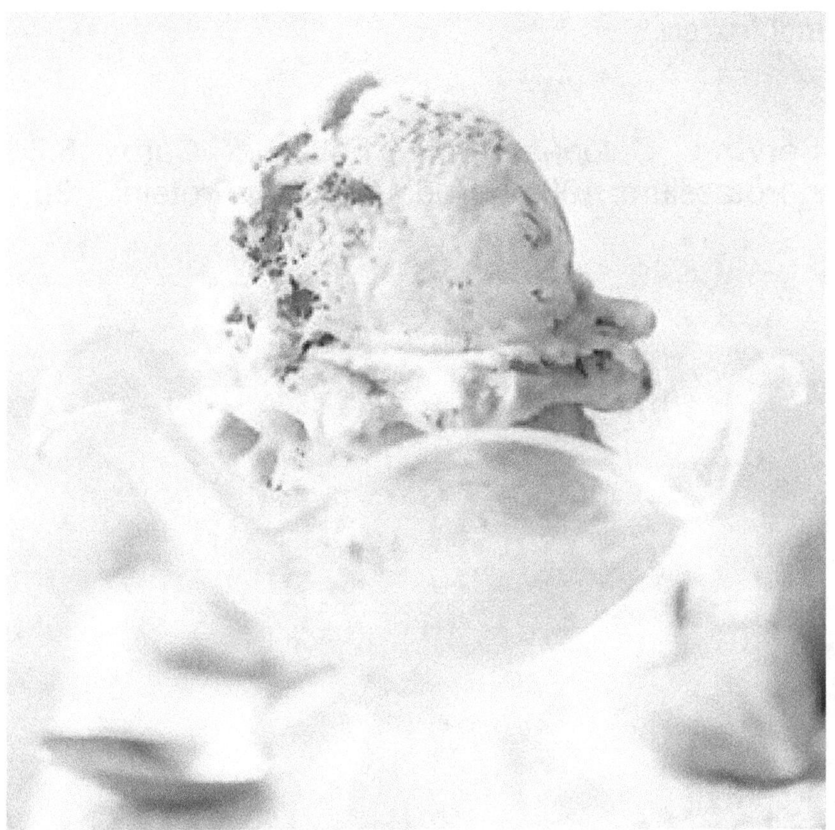

Preparation time: 5 minutes
Cooking time: 5 minutes
Servings: 3
Ingredients

- Stevia – ½ cup
- Lemon juice – 1 Tbsp.
- Non-dairy coffee creamer – ¾ cup
- Strawberries – 10 oz.
- Crushed ice – 1 cup

Direction:

1. Blend everything in a blend until smooth.

2. Freeze until frozen.
3. Serve.

Nutrition Per Serving Calories: 94.4 Fat: 6g Carb: 8.3g
Phosphorus: 25mg Potassium: 108mg Sodium: 25mg Protein: 1.3g

148. Cinnamon Custard

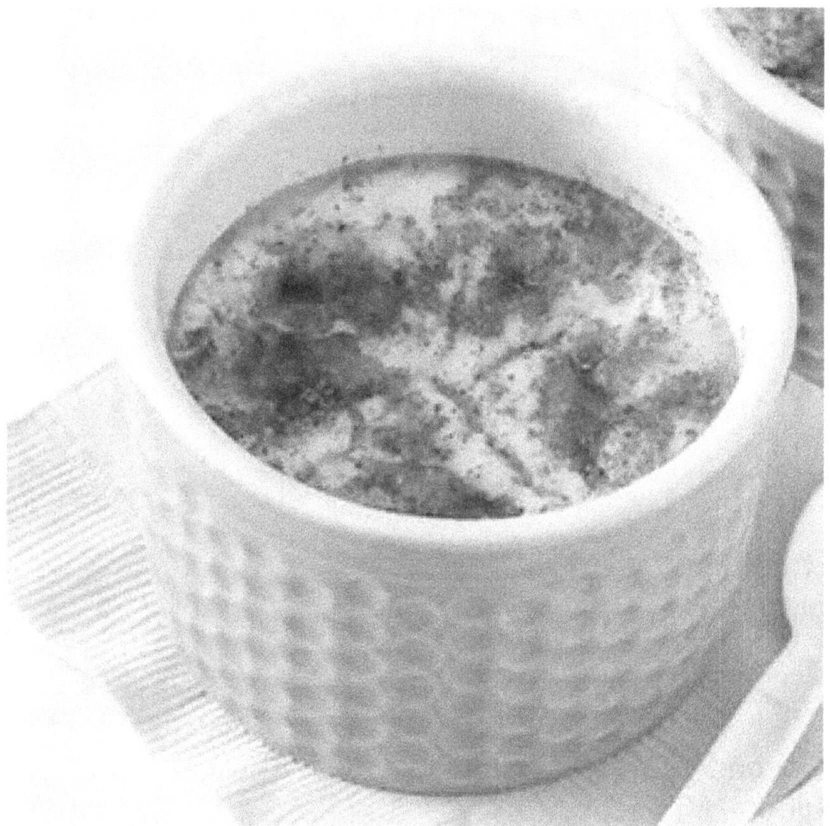

Preparation time: 20 minutes
Cooking time: 1 hour
Servings: 6
Ingredients

- Unsalted butter, for greasing the ramekins
- Plain rice milk – 1 ½ cups

- Eggs – 4
- Granulated sugar – ¼ cup
- Pure vanilla extract – 1 tsp.
- Ground cinnamon – ½ tsp.
- Cinnamon sticks for garnish

Direction:

1. Preheat the oven to 325F.
2. Lightly grease 6 ramekins and place them in a baking dish. Set aside.
3. In a large bowl, whisk together the eggs, rice milk, sugar, vanilla, and cinnamon until the mixture is very smooth.
4. Pour the mixture through a fine sieve into a pitcher.
5. Evenly divide the custard mixture among the ramekins.
6. Fill the baking dish with hot water, until the water reaches halfway up the sides of the ramekins.
7. Bake for 1 hour or until the custards are set and a knife inserted in the center comes out clean.
8. Remove the custards from the oven and take the ramekins out of the water.
9. Cool on the wire racks for 1 hour then chill for 1 hour.
10. Garnish with cinnamon sticks and serve.

Nutrition Per Serving Calories: 110 Fat: 4g Carb: 14g Phosphorus: 100mg Potassium: 64mg Sodium: 71mg Protein: 4g

149. Raspberry Brûlée

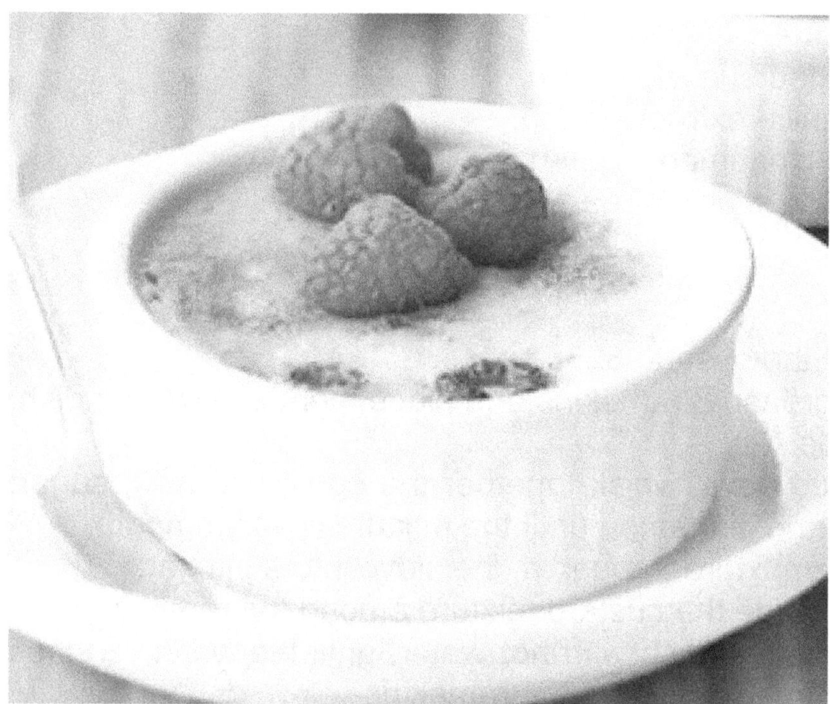

Preparation time: 15 minutes
Cooking time: 1 minutes
Servings: 4
Ingredients

- Light sour cream – ½ cup
- Plain cream cheese – ½ cup
- Brown sugar – ¼ cup, divided
- Ground cinnamon – ¼ tsp.
- Fresh raspberries – 1 cup

Direction:

1. Preheat the oven to broil.
2. In a bowl, beat together the cream cheese, sour cream, 2 tbsp. brown sugar and cinnamon for 4 minutes or until the mixture is very smooth and fluffy.

3. Evenly divide the raspberries among 4 (4-ounce) ramekins.
4. Spoon the cream cheese mixture over the berries and smooth the tops.
5. Sprinkle ½ tbsp. brown sugar evenly over each ramekin.
6. Place the ramekins on a baking sheet and broil 4 inches from the heating element until the sugar is caramelized and golden brown.
7. Cool and serve.

Nutrition Per Serving Calories: 188 Fat: 13g Carb: 16g Phosphorus: 60mg Potassium: 158mg Sodium: 132mg Protein: 3g

150. Peach Pecan Crisp

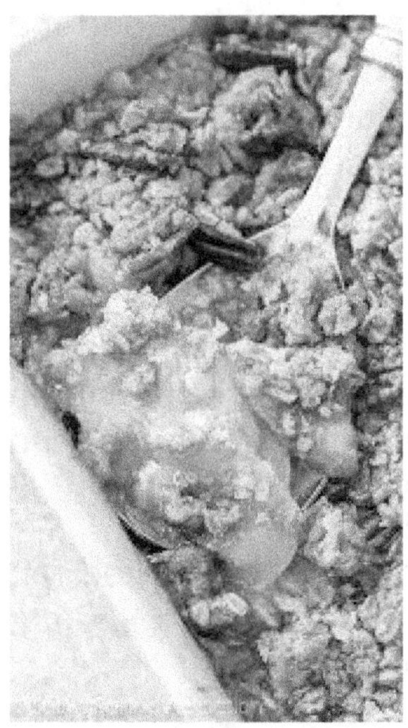

Preparation Time: 20 minutes
Cooking Time: 30 minutes
Serving: 8
Ingredients:

- Olive oil cooking spray
- 1½ cups rolled oats, divided
- 8 tablespoons brown sugar, divided
- 1/3 cup chopped pecans
- 1/4 cup butter, melted
- 4 peaches, peeled and sliced

Direction:

1. 1.Preheat the oven to 350°F. Spray a 9-inch square baking dish with cooking spray and set aside.
2. 2.In a large bowl, pour 1¼ cups of oats and set aside.
3. 3.In a food processor, place the remaining ¼ cup of oats and process until fine. Add to the rolled oats and mix.
4. 4.Add 6 tablespoons of brown sugar, the pecans, and the butter to the oat mixture and mix until crumbly.
5. 5.Combine the peaches and remaining 2 tablespoons of brown sugar in the prepared baking dish. Top with the oat mixture.
6. 6.Bake for 25 to 30 minutes, or until the peaches are bubbling and the streusel is golden brown. Let cool for 20 minutes, then serve.
7. Ingredient Tip: Simple swaps can make this recipe vegan and gluten-free. Replacing the butter with vegan butter and the oats with gluten-free oats is all that is needed.

Nutrition Per Serving Calories: 203; Total fat: 10g; Saturated fat: 4g; Sodium: 49mg; Phosphorus: 92mg; Potassium: 230mg; Carbohydrates: 27g; Fiber: 3g; Protein: 3g; Sugar: 15g

151. Peanut Butter Chocolate Fudge

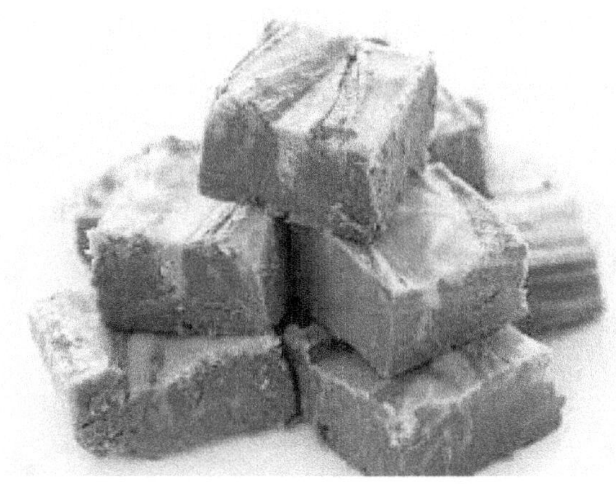

Preparation Time: 5 minutes
Cooking Time: 5 minutes
Serving: 18 pieces
Ingredients:

- 1 (12-ounce) package 60 percent (or higher) cacao chocolate chips
- 1/3 cup peanut butter
- 1 tablespoon butter

Direction:

1. 1.Line an 8-inch square baking dish with parchment paper and set aside.
2. 2.In a medium microwave-safe bowl, combine the chocolate chips, peanut butter, and butter. Microwave on 70 percent power for 1 minute; remove and stir. Continue microwaving for 30-second intervals, stirring each time, until the mixture is melted and smooth.
3. 3.Pour into the prepared pan and smooth the top.
4. 4.Refrigerate the fudge for 1 hour. Store for up to 5 days, covered, at room temperature.
5. Appliance Tip: You can make this recipe on the stovetop. Just combine the ingredients in a medium-size heavy

saucepan and melt over low heat, stirring frequently, until the mixture is melted and smooth.

Nutrition Per Serving (1 piece) Calories: 143; Total fat: 10g; Saturated fat: 5g; Sodium: 27mg; Phosphorus: 65mg; Potassium: 134mg; Carbohydrates: 11g; Fiber: 2g; Protein: 2g; Sugar: 7g

152. Rice Pudding with Raspberry Sauce

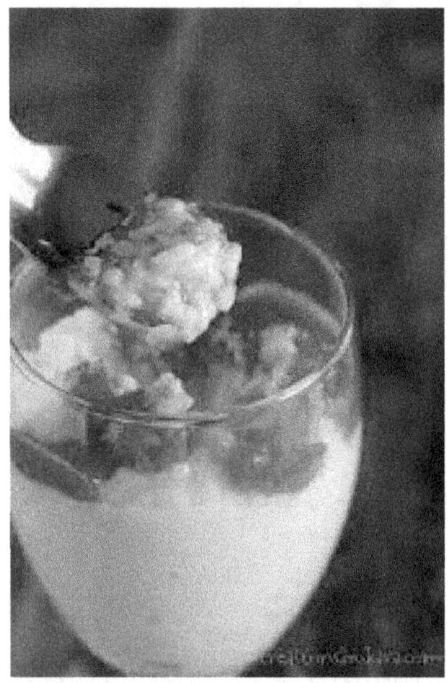

Preparation Time: 5 minutes
Cooking Time: 3 hours
Serving: 6
Ingredients:

- 2 cups unsweetened vanilla almond milk
- ½ cup white rice
- 1/3 cup sugar
- 1/8 teaspoon salt
- 2 ounces cream cheese, at room temperature
- 1 (10-ounce) bag frozen raspberries, thawed

Direction:

1. 1.In a 3-quart slow cooker, combine the almond milk, rice, sugar, and salt. Cover and cook on low for 2 hours. Cooking on high will make the rice cook unevenly.
2. 2.Stir the pudding, cover again, and cook for another 1 to 1½ hours or until the rice is very tender.
3. 3.Stir in the cream cheese until melted.
4. 4.Transfer to a bowl and place in the refrigerator until the rice pudding is chilled.
5. 5.In a blender or food processor, place the raspberries and blend until smooth. Pour into a bowl.
6. 6.You can serve the rice pudding after it's cooled, about 30 minutes. If you serve it cold, stir it again and serve with the raspberry sauce. Cover and store the raspberry sauce up to 3 days in the fridge.
7. Ingredient Tip: Feel free to try this rice pudding with brown rice. The cook time will change from 3 hours to 4 hours.

Nutrition Per Serving Calories: 169; Total fat: 5g; Saturated fat: 2g; Sodium: 140mg; Phosphorus: 50mg; Potassium: 171mg; Carbohydrates: 30g; Fiber: 2g; Protein: 3g; Sugar: 15g

153. No-Cook Velvety Cheesecake Parfaits

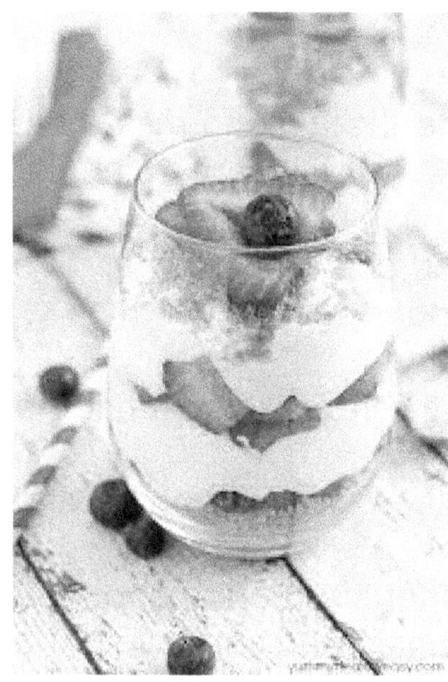

Preparation Time: 20 minutes
Cooking time: 0 minutes
Serving: 4
Ingredients:

- 1 (8-ounce) package cream cheese, at room temperature
- 1/3 cup powdered sugar
- ½ cup heavy cream
- 1 teaspoon vanilla extract
- 1½ cups chopped strawberries

Direction:

1. 1.In a medium bowl using a hand mixer on medium, beat the cream cheese and the powdered sugar until soft and well-blended.
2. 2.In a small bowl using the mixer on high, beat the cream and vanilla for 4 to 6 minutes, until soft peaks form. Fold the whipped cream into the cream cheese mixture.

3. 3.Into glasses, layer the cream cheese mixture with the strawberries. For an extra-fancy presentation, use parfait or stemmed glasses. Cover and chill for 2 to 3 hours before serving.
4. Diabetes Tip: To make this recipe diabetes-friendly, omit the powdered sugar and replace with 1/3 cup plus 2 tablespoons of powdered erythritol. The carbohydrate content will decrease to 9g.

Nutrition Per Serving Calories: 359; Total fat: 30g; Saturated fat: 18g; Sodium: 187mg; Phosphorus: 92mg; Potassium: 192mg; Carbohydrates: 18g; Fiber: 1g; Protein: 5g; Sugar: 16g

154. Peanut Butter Coconut Bars

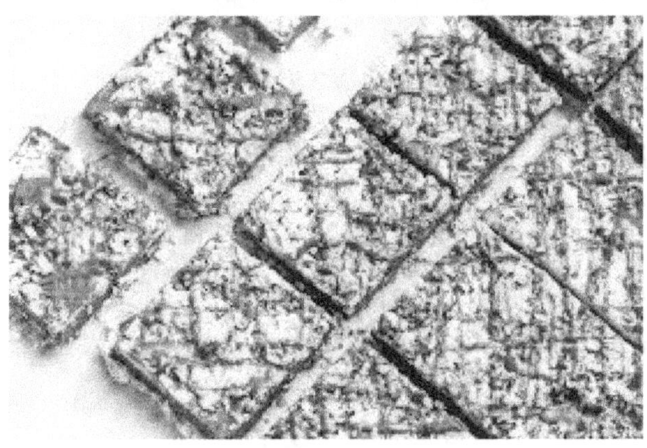

Preparation Time: 10 minutes
Cooking Time: 5 minutes, plus 3 hours to set
Serving: 25 bars
Ingredients:

- 1¼ cups peanut butter, divided
- ½ cup honey
- 1¼ cups graham cracker crumbs
- 1 cup unsweetened shredded coconut flakes
- 1 cup 60 percent cacao chocolate chips

Direction:

1. 1.In a large saucepan, combine 1 cup of peanut butter and the honey over medium heat. Melt, stirring frequently.
2. 2.Add the graham cracker crumbs and coconut and stir until combined. Press into an 8-inch square pan.
3. 3.In a small microwave-safe bowl, combine the remaining ¼ cup of peanut butter and the chocolate chips. Microwave on high for 30 seconds; remove and stir. Continue microwaving for 30-second intervals, stirring after each interval, until the mixture is smooth.
4. 4.Pour over the bars and let stand for 3 hours to cool and set.
5. 5.When cool, cut into 5 strips and then cut those strips into 5.
6. Ingredient Tip: This recipe would also work with other nut and seed butters such as almond butter and sunflower seed butter.

Nutrition Per Serving (1 bar) Calories: 179; Total fat: 12g; Saturated fat: 5g; Sodium: 79mg; Phosphorus: 77mg; Potassium: 141mg; Carbohydrates: 16g; Fiber: 2g; Protein: 4g; Sugar: 11g

155. Mixed Berry Fruit Salad

Preparation Time: 20 minutes
Cooking time: 0 minutes
Serving: 4
Ingredients:

- 1½ cups raspberries, divided
- 1½ cups sliced strawberries
- 1 cup blackberries
- 1/3 cup sour cream
- 1 tablespoon chopped fresh mint leaves

Direction:

1. 1.In a medium bowl, combine 1¼ cups of raspberries with the strawberries and blackberries and mix gently.
2. 2.In a small bowl, place the remaining ¼ cup of raspberries and crush with a fork. Stir in the sour cream and mint leaves.
3. 3.Divide into serving cups, top with the sour cream mixture, and serve.
4. Make It Easier Tip: Instead of the chopped fresh mint leaves, you can add a few drops of mint extract to the sour cream. It's easy to go overboard, so add the extract just a drop at a time and taste as you go.

Nutrition Per Serving Calories: 95; Total fat: 4g; Saturated fat: 2g; Sodium: 7mg; Phosphorus: 49mg; Potassium: 239mg; Carbohydrates: 14g; Fiber: 6g; Protein: 2g; Sugar: 7g

156. Peach-Filled Meringue

Preparation Time: 40 minutes
Cooking Time: 1 hour
Serving: 6
Ingredients:

- 4 large egg whites
- 1 cup powdered sugar
- 2 teaspoons freshly squeezed lemon juice, divided
- ½ cup heavy whipping cream
- 4 fresh peaches, peeled and chopped

Direction:

1. 1.Preheat the oven to 350°F. Line a baking sheet with parchment paper and set aside.

2. 2.The egg whites should be at room temperature, so let them stand for 20 minutes after you have separated them.
3. 3.Once the egg whites are at room temperature, place them into a bowl and using a hand mixer on high, beat for about 3 minutes, until peaks begin to form. Beat in the powdered sugar 2 tablespoons at a time for about 3 to 5 minutes longer.
4. 4.Fold in 1 teaspoon of lemon juice.
5. 5.To keep the parchment paper from sliding off the baking sheet, dab a bit of the meringue on the bottom side and put back onto the baking sheet.
6. 6.Form 6 small circles of the meringue, about 4 inches across and 1 inch thick, on the parchment paper.
7. 7.Place in the oven and reduce the heat immediately to 300°F. Bake for 1 hour, then turn off the heat, open the oven door slightly, and let the meringues cool.
8. 8.In a medium bowl and using a hand mixer on high, beat the cream for 4 to 6 minutes, until soft peaks form. Fold in the remaining 1 teaspoon of lemon juice and the peaches.
9. 9.Turn the little meringues over and top with the cream mixture. Cover and refrigerate for 2 to 3 hours, then serve.

10. Ingredient Tip: It's easier to separate egg whites from the yolks while the egg is cold. Crack the egg and gently pry the two halves of the shell open. Over a small bowl, rock the yolk from one shell to the other until all the egg white is in the bowl. Transfer the white to a large bowl for beating and repeat. Let stand for at least 20 minutes after separating to reach room temperature.

Nutrition Per Serving Calories: 196; Total fat: 7g; Saturated fat: 5g; Sodium: 43mg; Phosphorus: 34mg; Potassium: 247mg; Carbohydrates: 30g; Fiber: 2g; Protein: 4g; Sugar: 29g

157. Filo Apple Hand Pies

Preparation Time: 25 minutes
Cooking Time: 25 minutes
Serving: 8
Ingredients:

- 1 medium Granny Smith apple, peeled and chopped
- ¼ cup sugar
- 6 tablespoons butter, divided
- 1 teaspoon vanilla extract
- 8 (9-by-14-inch) filo sheets, thawed

Direction:

1. 1.In a medium saucepan, combine the apples, sugar, and 2 tablespoons of butter. Bring to a simmer over medium heat, then reduce heat to low and simmer for 5 to 7 minutes or until the apples are tender. Transfer to a bowl and place in the freezer to cool for 30 minutes.
2. 2.Remove the apple mixture from the freezer, add the vanilla, and stir.
3. 3.Preheat the oven to 350°F.
4. 4.In a small saucepan, melt the remaining 4 tablespoons of butter and pour into a small bowl.
5. 5.Place one of the filo sheets on the work surface and brush with a bit of the butter. Layer one more sheet onto the first sheet.
6. 6.Fold the filo stack in half to make a 4½-by-14-inch rectangle. Put 2 to 3 tablespoons of the apple mixture on the end of the strip. Fold the bottom right corner up to the left side so the bottom becomes the left side, then fold straight. Bring the bottom left corner up to the right side and fold straight. Seal the pastry with a bit of butter and place on a baking sheet.

7. 7.Repeat with the remaining filo, butter, and apple filling. Brush all the pastries with the remaining butter.
8. 8.Bake for 15 to 20 minutes or until the filo is crisp and golden brown. Remove to a cooling rack to cool and set aside.
9. Make It Easier Tip: You can assemble these little pies up to 8 hours ahead of time and then put them in the fridge. When you're ready, bake as directed, adding a few minutes of baking time for the cold pies.
10. Ingredient Tip: You can refreeze filo dough. Just wrap it in the original wrapping, put it back into the box, seal the box with tape, and freeze. You can also freeze the little pies once they are completely cool.

Nutrition Per Serving (1 hand pie) Calories: 236; Total fat: 9g; Saturated fat: 5g; Sodium: 168mg; Phosphorus: 39mg; Potassium: 59mg; Carbohydrates: 35g; Fiber: 1g; Protein: 4g; Sugar: 9g

158. Watermelon Mint Granita

Preparation Time: 15 minutes, plus 2 hours to chill
Cooking time: 0 minutes
Serving: 4
Ingredients:

- 4 cups watermelon cubes, seeded
- ¼ cup sugar
- 2 tablespoons freshly squeezed lemon juice
- 2 tablespoons minced fresh mint leaves

Direction:

1. 1.In a blender or food processor, combine the watermelon, sugar, lemon juice, and mint and blend until smooth.

2. 2.Pour the mixture into a 9-inch square pan. Freeze for 2 hours, stirring the mixture once during freezing time.
3. 3.To serve, scrape up some of the granita with a fork and spoon lightly into glasses.
4. Make It Easier Tip: Buy seedless watermelon and you won't have to remove the seeds. There are still seeds in seedless watermelon, but they are so small and tender you can eat them.

NutritionPer Serving Calories: 81; Total fat: 0g; Saturated fat: 0g; Sodium: 1mg; Phosphorus: 12mg; Potassium: 123mg; Carbohydrates: 21g; Fiber: 0g; Protein: 1g; Sugar: 19g

159. Peanut Butter Mug Cake

Preparation Time: 5 minutes
Cooking Time: 2 minutes
Serving: 1
Ingredients:

- 3 tablespoons gluten-free flour blend
- 2 tablespoons peanut butter
- 2 tablespoons almond milk
- 4 teaspoons brown sugar
- ¼ teaspoon Low-Phosphorus Baking Powder

Direction:

1. 1.In an 8-ounce microwave-safe mug, combine the flour blend, peanut butter, almond milk, brown sugar, and baking powder and stir until combined.
2. 2.Microwave on high for 45 to 60 seconds or until the cake springs back when lightly touched with a finger. If the cake isn't done, microwave for 10-second intervals until it does spring back.

3. 3.Let cool for 3 to 4 minutes and eat.
4. Ingredient Tip: Stir in 1 tablespoon of chocolate chips before cooking this little cake for a Chocolate Peanut Butter Mug Cake.

Nutrition Per Serving (1 cake) Calories: 482; Total fat: 28g; Saturated fat: 7g; Sodium: 230mg; Phosphorus: 217mg; Potassium: 384mg; Carbohydrates: 48g; Fiber: 3g; Protein: 14g; Sugar: 24g

Volume Equivalents (Liquid)

1. US STANDARD	US STANDARD (OZ.)	METRIC (APPROXIMATE)
2 tbsp.	1 fl. oz.	30 mL
1/4 cup	2 fl. oz.	60 mL
1/2 cup	4 fl. oz.	120 mL
1 cup	8 fl. oz.	240 mL
11/2 cups	12 fl. oz.	355 mL
2 cups or 1 pint	16 fl. oz.	475 mL
4 cups or 1 quart	32 fl. oz.	1 L
1 gallon	128 fl. oz.	4 L

Volume Equivalents (Dry)

US STANDARD	METRIC (APPROXIMATE)
1/4 tsp.	1 mL
1/2 tsp.	2 mL
1 tsp.	5 mL
1 tbsp.	15 mL
1/4 cup	59 mL
cup	79 mL

1/2 cup	118 mL
1 cup	177 mL

Weight Equivalents

US STANDARD	METRIC (APPROXIMATE)
1/2 oz.	15 g
1 oz.	30 g
2 oz.	60 g
4 oz.	115 g
8 oz.	225 g
12 oz.	340 g
16 oz. or 1 lb.	455 g

Oven Temperatures

FAHRENHEIT (F)	CELSIUS (C) (APPROXIMATE)
250°F	120 °C
300°F	150°C
325°F	165°C
350°F	180°C
375°F	190°C
400°F	200°C
425°F	220°C
450°F	230°C

www.ingramcontent.com/pod-product-compliance
Lightning Source LLC
Chambersburg PA
CBHW080718260726
48660CB00010B/3585